THERE'S THE LIGHTHOUSE

There's the Lighthouse. 'We're almost there.'
'He's doing very well,' said Macalister,
praising James. 'He's keeping her very steady.'

To the Lighthouse by Virginia Woolf

The trouble with Adrian (and later with Karin) was pretty complicated and dated from prehistoric childhood. Some of it is used in James in *To the Lighthouse.*

A letter from Leonard Woolf to his niece,
Adrian Stephen's daughter, Ann.

By the same author

When the Weather's Changing (*Novel*)

I Meant to Marry Him (*Autobiography*)

Books for young people, including

Hal
Liz
Jobs for the Girls
Three's Company
A Special Providence
The Spy in Dolor Hugo

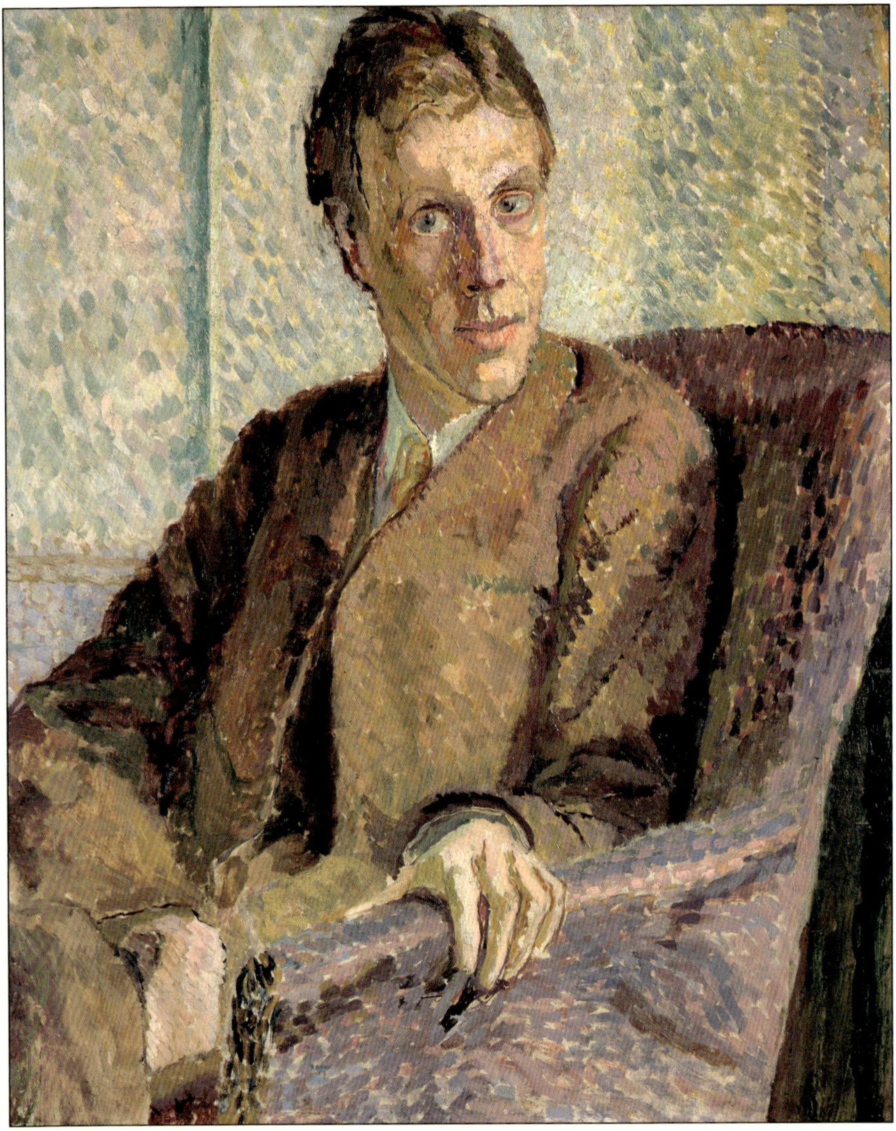

A portrait of Adrian Stephen by Duncan Grant

THERE'S THE LIGHTHOUSE

A Biography of Adrian Stephen

Jean MacGibbon

JAMES
X
JAMES

First published 1997

ISBN 0 907 383 769

Designed by
Oliver Hickey

Printed in Great Britain
by Butler & Tanner Ltd

Published by James & James (Publishers) Ltd
Gordon House Business Centre
6 Lissenden Garden
London NW5 1LX

PUBLISHER'S FOREWORD

Quentin Bell favoured a biography being written of his uncle, Adrian Stephen, of whom he was fond. When a new edition of Adrian's account of the Dreadnought Hoax came out long after his death he wrote an admiring introduction. He and Olivier Bell encouraged the author from the start, providing valuable information and anecdotes and constructive comments. He seemed pleased with Adrian's professional status, as a man in his own right outside Bloomsbury although he was 'of it but not in it' – as Desmond MacCarthy described his own association with the group of friends. Quentin Bell told the author, for instance, that Adrian had told him that Lytton Strachey and other Apostles were shocked by Adrian's complete rejection of G. E. Moore. 'To some extent he was advancing views which were accepted by many people but not at that time, and in fact was fighting a kind of one-man battle against that generation at Cambridge.' Shortly before his death, after he had read the final draft, he undertook to write a foreword but alas! it was too late. With the approval of Olivier Bell extracts from two letters he wrote to the author follow.

In April 1996, after reading an early, unedited part of the typescript: 'I could not resist reading the first 44 pages of Adrian this morning. I reminded myself that this is an early draft . . . and I must admit that I used my pedantic pencil a great deal. Then, after a few pages the prose clarified, it became easy, indeed delightful reading and although there was very little I didn't know already I forged ahead most happily and with admiration. I like it very much.'

After reading the final draft in September 1996: 'I do like it, it is a very good read and also I think a good likeness, also I think a good likeness of Karin, a most unhappy woman.' (In both letters he made constructive comments, such as there being more than necessary about the Stephen family and that the Cambridge chapter might be extended. All his comments and Olivier Bell's exhaustive corrections of detail have of course been incorporated.)

CONTENTS

LIST OF PLATES

ACKNOWLEDGEMENTS

My thanks are due, first and foremost, to the late Professor Quentin Bell and to Mrs Olivier Bell, whose warm friendship and his favourable reception to the idea of a book about his uncle, have been the happiest experience of our joint labours – my husband's and mine – during the past six years. They were both of the greatest help to me with advice and information, checking the text and permission to quote from his biography of Virginia Woolf and many letters. Our dear friend Frances Partridge also read the MS and gave invaluable help throughout as the oldest surviving friend of Adrian and what are loosely called 'the Bloomsbury Group'.

Ann Synge, like a true Stephen, 'didn't much favour a book about her father but wouldn't hinder me', and dispatched an elderly but distinguished-looking battered leather suitcase which proved to contain the material, got together by Adrian's second daughter, the late Judith Henderson, on which much of this book is based. Richard Holmes gave valuable time and friendship to a constructive reorganisation of the MS. Antonia Till, my editor, brought an experienced and critical talent to improving, every step of the way, a book too hastily thrown together against time and old age. The late Nonie Wintour gave discriminating attention to the MS, reading it chapter by chapter until her death. Athol Hughes, analyst and writer, introduced me to analysts who might help me. Pearl King, another analyst and writer, retired deputy archivist of the British Psychoanalytical Society, allowed me to quote extracts from *The Freud–Klein Controversies 1941–1945* jointly edited by her and Ricardo Steiner, and gave me general advice. Sir Benedict Hoskyns advised me on medical matters. Conan Nicholas edited the text in detail, read the proofs and compiled the index with consummate professionalism and understanding of the subject matter; any errors remaining being entirely mine.

Personal memories have been contributed by Adrian and Karin's surviving patients: Malcolm Pines, whose knowledge of early analysts was invaluable; Lord Young of Dartington and my cousin,

Elizabeth Jane Howard, novelist and critic; Marion Milner, writer and analyst, and a close friend of Adrian and Karin, was helpful and so was her niece, Giovanna Bloor, who gave me her child's-eye view of the King's Head. Yvonne Kapp is another patient who was of the greatest help. Mrs Patrick Evans, whose father, Lt.-Col. Richard Rendell was a great friend of Adrian, gave me a helpful interview. Barbara Halpern Strachey has been a ready source of information about the Stephen family and allowed me to quote from her book and to keep for many months her index of Karin's letters to her mother, Mary Berenson, which was indispensable in defining a framework of time and place to the book. Jane Dunn's *A Very Close Relationship* was of great use to me as was Noël Annan's *Leslie Stephen.* Richard Shone was specially generous with his assistance.

Richard Garnett allowed me to quote a passage from *The Golden Echo* by his father, David Garnett and his letter to Anne Olivier Bell. I acknowledge with many thanks the permission given to me by the Manuscripts Section of the University of Sussex library and Elizabeth Inglis and the late Trekie Parsons to quote from Leonard Woolf's books and his letter to Ann Synge. I also thank Michael Holroyd for permission to quote from his biography of Lytton Strachey. For permission to quote Betty Miller's to-the-life portrait of Adrian Stephen in her novel, *On the Side of the Angels*, and her letter to Sir John Verney, I am specially grateful to her daughter, Sarah Miller. The Society of Authors, the literary representative of the Estate of Virginia Woolf, kindly allowed me to quote from her novel, *To The Lighthouse*, and her many observations of her brother in her Diaries and Letters, on which much of my narrative depends. The Record Office, Ministry of Defence, even while their premises were being reconstructed, gave me a complete record of Adrian's army career. Henrietta Garnett allowed me to quote two letters of Duncan Grant and to reproduce his portrait of Adrian and for this I am grateful. The two letters of J. M. Keynes to Duncan Grant are from The Unpublished Writings of J. M. Keynes, copyright the Provost and Scholars of King's College, Cambridge 1997. I copied them from Robert Skidelsky's biography of J. M. Keynes and I acknowledge with many thanks the permission given to me by the Provost and Scholars of King's College, Cambridge to quote them.

Other individuals have helped me in a variety of ways: Marjorie Beadle; Dr Cook, School of Tropical Medicine; Gwenda David; Professor Samuel Hynes, Princeton University; Mervyn Jones; Mrs L. A. Rhodes, the Cremation Society; Dr George Rylands; Robert

Skidelsky; Frances Spalding; Judge Stephen Sedley; and special thanks to Susan Watson for her early memories of Adrian and Karin and their daughters.

Archivists and librarians at the following all gave me generously of their time and skill: King's College, Trinity College, and Newnham College, Cambridge; the University of Sussex; the Wellcome Institute for the History of Medicine; the Tate Gallery; the Lilly Library, University of Indiana; the Hertfordshire County Library; the Uxbridge Central Library. For special assistance I am indebted to Professor Hugh Brogan, the University of Essex, who handed me over to Jean Cropton, the assistant archivist, without whose help in deciphering the film of Karin Stephen's American letters, an important source, would have been denied me.

Without Dr Leslie Sohn's long and patient analysis neither this nor any other of my books could have been written. It is customary to acknowledge the exemplary devotion shown by spouses to wayward writers. But James did more, helping me with my researches, typing the first fair copy and making resumés of *The Dreadnought Hoax* and, saving me many hours of reading, *The Controversial Discussions.*

Jean MacGibbon
Keats Grove,
London, May 1997

CHAPTER 1

PROLOGUE

We first met Adrian and Karin Stephen in 1942 through Julian Trevelyan, the painter, then one of the camouflage officers at VIII Corps Headquarters near Taunton, along with James, my husband who was an Intelligence Officer. The occasion was the regular *thé dansant* at the County Hotel organised to while away officers' idle Sunday afternoons. A more incongruous meeting-place can hardly be imagined. Adrian and Karin were, in their way, even more striking than Julian himself. Adrian was six feet five inches tall, his height emphasised by his gaunt physique. Karin's commanding presence gave an impression of height, her high colour contrasting with his clear pallor, her blazing blue eyes surveying the dancers, marking down Bernard Floud, James's fellow intelligence officer. Adrian's lighter blue eyes were disconcerting in their enquiring candour. James told me afterwards that Karin was not a good dancer, with little sense of rhythm, and masterful, always wanting to 'lead'.

But away she went with Bernard at the first opportunity, he restrained, correct, upright, as though modestly conscious of being the best dancer on the floor. 'He had lessons from Santos Casani,'[1] I said. 'He would,' said James sourly.

Adrian put back his head and laughed quietly, a laugh that was to become familiar, for we got to know one another that afternoon among the tea-cups, the cake-stands, the dainty silver forks. In the interval a black sergeant from one of the nearby military battalion bands played Bach and jazz superbly, privately to himself, across the empty floor.

Adrian did not dance. So we talked, or, for the most part, I talked and he listened, with an attentiveness that both alarmed and entranced me. Alarmed, perhaps, because I had been told he was a

1 Well-known dancing instructor

psychoanalyst, a profession I then associated with witchcraft. Entranced, because his appearance and his manner, simple and direct as it was, gave me the feeling that I was in the presence of someone unique, larger than life.

He had a kind of beauty rather than handsomeness. His fine-boned features, his expressive mouth, gentle humour, quick response, and his voice, musical, quiet, but not low-pitched – all made their mark on me.

I asked him what he did and he told me he was a psychiatrist in the RAMC working in a military hospital at Lydeard St Lawrence treating casualties from Dunkirk. 'Too late', he said, 'to be of any use. They should have been seen at once, not six months or more after the event.'

Julian had told me that Adrian was Virginia Woolf's brother. I knew little about her or her background. I had given up reading her books towards the end of the Thirties, for reading her was pure pleasure which I felt to be wrong when our world was on the edge of destruction. When Hitler marched into Austria I broke my favourite Richard Strauss record over my knee and buried Virginia in a tea-chest. If this seems exaggerated, Adrian himself told me that the first time he put on his hated battledress he determined to wear it until the war's end, even on leave.

I rather brashly asked him if he had come into any of Virginia Woolf's novels? He answered flatly in his reticent way, 'I was the boy who wanted to go to the lighthouse.'[2]

I had begun to feel unwell and, without a word, went to the lavatory, then asked James to take me home. I wrote to Adrian apologising, writing that I must have been stiff and unnatural, as though wearing a 'jet corsage'. He wrote back that anything less like a 'jet corsage' would be hard to imagine. He was curious; we had, he felt, been getting on rather well. Then I had suddenly asked James to take me home. Why, he wondered? We met again, but I remember only a number of us sitting in a pub in Taunton while the Stephens' daughter Judith played a fruit machine with Bernard. Then Adrian and Karin moved away.

We occasionally corresponded, though if one of the purposes of letter-writing is for the writers to get to know each other better, I doubt if we did. Adrian, as I was to discover later when we were able to meet, was sometimes chillingly reticent and disliked talking and writing about himself. My letters were muddled, basically insincere and not really about myself, which might have interested him.

[2] *To The Lighthouse*, Virginia Woolf, 1927.

I used them to practise writing. His answers were short but carefully considered. When I asked him why he took so much trouble, he answered simply, 'I've taken to you.'

Adrian was fond of young women – tender and amused, attentive when they were in trouble. I had written to him about one of these entanglements brought about by war, instability and absence. Towards the end of the summer in 1942 an opportunity occurred for me to spend a night or two with James, now at the War Office in one of the sections dealing with preparations for D-Day.

We met Adrian at St Pancras Station, where James left us. 'I had the feeling he was handing me over to you,' Adrian said later. In Regent's Park I sat on a grassy knoll, my back against a tree, my striped cotton skirt outspread, white net gloves on my lap, tears rolling down my cheeks. 'It's not that I mind, it's over. It's just that I am tired – so tired.'

He lay on the grass, leaning on his elbow, his whole length stretched out, his wide blue eyes attentive. There wasn't much to be said. But I felt released from the obsession, the humiliation, the sordidness of the affair I had come to talk to him about. It was indeed ended. Lightheartedly, we walked by the lake that warm summer evening, barrage balloons up in a lightly clouded sky the only sign of war. We ate in a café and I saw him back to the station. 'I nearly kissed you then,' he told me later. For my part, I had fallen deeply, disastrously, in love.

We did not meet again for over a year, in a top-floor flat whither I had crazily moved with the children, Hamish nine, Janet seven, uprooting us from a secure haven in a farmhouse near Taunton where they were cared for by the farmer's wife, who became a friend for life, so that I could get on with my novel (I had had two short stories published by John Lehmann in Folios of New Writing and in Penguin New Writing).

Such was our faith in Marshal Zhukov and the Russian Army that, though they were still hard-pressed by the Germans before Stalingrad, it seemed safe to start another child and by the end of August I was pregnant. I wanted to have our baby in London; and to be near James. I think now that, paradoxically, it was partly because of my love for Adrian, of which James knew nothing. Had it been simply an 'affair', affairs were common enough in wartime. What made me anxious and guilty was my loving him so much.

When he came that first time to Westbourne Terrace, for a while we said nothing. He sat on the sofa, his head bowed, his fingers interlocked in front of him. I knelt at his feet and hit his wrists with the sides of my hands in a rabbit punch, breaking his grip. We kissed and I lay in his arms.

There were few more such meetings; once we walked in Kensington Gardens. He told me about his family, and recounted legends about their past. He liked to imitate people in his stories. He re-enacted the one about his great-uncle who had died in India, his body packed in spirit in a barrel. When it was deposited in the hall, in London, the barrel burst open and the corpse arose. The story is famous; but I doubt if it was ever more graphically told than by Adrian, rising slowly to his full height, deathly pale.

He described the house they went to whenever he had leave, on an Essex estuary, full of islands, channels and little creeks. From here he and Karin sailed out to the open sea, sometimes to France or Holland. Once he wrote from there, 'there is a tearing wind over the marshes.'

'What do you do when you can't sleep?' I asked.

'I navigate past the Kentish Knock.' This, I afterwards found, is a light vessel marking a sandbank in the Thames estuary.

Towards winter air-raids began again unexpectedly after a long pause. James was bunkered in the War Office. I found a torch, woke Hamish, and slung Janet still sleeping over my shoulder, urging Hamish down steep stairs till we found an alcove reasonably safe from breaking windows. Hamish stayed with Janet in the dark while I fetched a rug, drinks, games, books, biscuits and the inevitable enamel pot. This became a nightly picnic. But James, who knew of the imminent threat of a new German weapon, rockets fired from Holland, thought we were better out of London. We went to stay with friends, Dorry and Rupert Metcalf, in their cottage near Newdigate in Surrey.

Robert was born in April in a London nursing home. Three days later I bundled him into his carrycot and joined James and the children. He had been given ten days' compassionate leave to look after them. But Robert was born some days late and I was soon left to cope on my own.

Marelands, Rupert and Dorry's house, was ideal for children; they ran about the fields and woods and Hamish soon grew brown all over. Janet made friends with some Italian prisoners working in the fields. She climbed the hedge in her blue-checked gingham dress, guessing they were homesick. They gave her bacon sandwiches, a rare luxury; and one of them showed her a photograph of his own daughter back in Italy.

Robert was not so happy. He cried night and day till the district nurse came and gave him National Dried Milk to supplement my breast-feeding.

Dorry, an American, was determined to continue her education by correspondence course. She lay by the duck-pond, carefully tanning herself all over while reading her book on nineteenth-century economics. I lay beside her feeding Robert, his body close and warm beside mine. This must have been the most contented time of his babyhood. For I suffered acutely from post-natal depression, a condition not then recognised.

I went up to London with Robert in his carrycot to see Adrian. The second time I made importunate demands on him; kissing was not enough. He himself, I know now, was not well; his wife, a manic-depressive, was ill. And he was thirty years older than I.

'What difference would it make?'

'It would make all the difference.'

'You have made me miserable,' he said, with his head in his hands, 'and that brat of yours is crying.'

Next day he wrote, 'If we had been married I think I could have made love to you as James never could, and as I never could to Karin. But we are not married.'

There were times, those summer evenings, when my feeling for James was as it had been, and Adrian seemed an unreal dream. I remember one such evening when James came down to see us. We lay close to one another under my school cloak in a westward-facing lean-to, my hand in his, comforting and secure. But 'as it had been' was not enough. There had been no solid building on our earlier, youthful love. True, we needed each other. But need alone isn't a good basis for marriage. And though there ran a deep spring, a hope for lasting love, through much that we did and felt, together and apart, for me this source of common sense and sanity, ultimately of moral sense, was running low.

Towards the end of August I had to undergo a serious abdominal operation. A nurse was found to take Robert; and leaving the other two with a friend, I entered University College Hospital. But the day before Hamish went down with appendicitis. I fetched him by ambulance and a bed was found for him in an amenity ward. Thus Janet was left alone with a strange woman, bereft of Hamish, her constant companion and source of security in James's absence, till my mother came and took her away.

Adrian came to see me in hospital, throwing off his army raincoat on the bed and unbuckling his Sam Browne belt, held me close. Afterwards he went and saw Hamish, who dimly remembers the apparition of a tall officer in an army raincoat.

My sister was given compassionate leave from the Navy to take the children for three months. For a fortnight Robert was sent to a baby's home run by a cousin. We went to see him. Sitting up in his cot, he looked up when the door was opened, looking not for us but for the nurse who had cared for him till she got ill. I have re-run that scene over and over again. Why did I not pick him up and take him home, to a ground-floor flat or a house, and keep him on my knee all day? We left him until a nurse could be found to look after him in the flat and I was well enough to take over.

For a year I stopped writing to Adrian, not wanting him to get mixed up in the crazy chaos that ensued. Eventually a school was found for Hamish and Janet, one founded for just such a plight as theirs, where Janet says they were happy and gained a sense of security and continuity.

A year later, in June 1944, James was posted to Washington, and I took Robert to Cornwall, to Cadgwith, a fishing-village near the tip of the Lizard, the only place where I could be sure of being fed, and give all my attention to restoring Robert's confidence. We lived with a fisherman's family, the Mitchells, who had children the same age as Hamish and Janet who came down for the holidays. By day, Robert and I spent our mornings on the beach in the little cove, Robert bringing me a pile of green, serpentine pebbles while I corrected the proofs of my novel, *When the Weather's Changing.* At night when he was in bed I sat in the lamplight reading books sent by the London Library.

The convoys escorted by the Royal Navy passed close by the Lizard; and when there was fog and the foghorn boomed its melancholy warning, a lurking German submarine would pick off one of our ships. Robert woke up and ran round his cot, thinking that the guns and the noise meant that we were to go down to an air-raid shelter. I took him into bed and together we slept.

I saw no one but the Mitchells; and wrote long letters to James. His were full of accounts of parties and people he was meeting. 'We went to St Elizabeth Hospital whose head, Tiny Zimon, gives marvellous parties. A long-haired girl played boogie-woogie on the harp and the sofa was covered in real fur.' He went to a waltz club on Saturday nights.

After the April holidays we all returned to London. I had begun to feel that there was too great a contrast between the life that suited me in Cornwall and the active social life James so obviously needed. At last I told him we must separate. For some twenty-four hours I was elated – I had done the right thing. Then – there is no word to describe it – I fell into a black hole, total breakdown. A friend came and took Robert. I wrote to James again saying I could not live without him. But he won't come, I thought; and Dr Joan Malleson whom I consulted thought so too. 'If he comes back he must have a fixation on you.'

Of all this James knew nothing but he had replied passionately telling me we must not separate. And it is at this point that Adrian took a hand. I had cut myself off from him and everyone else, including my mother. But Dr Malleson and he knew each other and she must have told him of her concern. He got in touch with the War Office, no doubt exploiting his high professional reputation. The first James heard about it was when he was called in by his brigadier: 'I am sorry to tell you your wife is very ill and I have arranged for you to return at once.' James was flown back in an RAF plane next day.

After the war we remained friends with them both. James saw another side of Adrian: he was a clubbable man. James wanted to join the Savile Club, and Adrian asked him to dinner to meet other members. James saw how well he was liked. It was the same I found when I began to write about him. His fellow analysts showed an equal regard for him, in contrast to Karin; her pushy, aggressive manner alienated them, in spite of her brilliant intellect, as it had Adrian's friends and family.

His heart trouble was worsening; and in October 1947 when we went to see him on his birthday his appearance was shocking. When we left, as we crossed the hall, he put an arm round my shoulder. 'You're a nice creature,' he said. This was almost the last time we saw him before his death in 1948.

Adrian Stephen never spoke about himself when we were together, and his reticence, then and now, both frustrated and fascinated me. He remained an enigma: what had formed this man, what influences and inheritance? What had led him to his demanding marriage and kept him within it in spite of difficulties and separations? What had attracted him to the new science of psychoanalysis? What, after the grievously premature death of his much loved elder brother, Thoby, had made Adrian feel that 'the wrong man died'? When, nearly fifty years after his death, I began to write about him I found him no less elusive, and felt somehow that he had deliberately covered his tracks. He wrote few letters except to his family and Duncan Grant, and he kept a diary only for a few months in 1909. Writing about him has been not so much a detective exercise as an attempt to lay hands on an animal for ever retreating into the undergrowth, slipping out of my grasp.

2

LESLIE AND JULIA

Adrian Leslie Stephen, the younger son of Leslie and Julia Stephen, was born on October 27, 1883 at 22 Hyde Park Gate, London. In the fourth-floor nursery he joined Vanessa (four), Julian Thoby (three) and Adeline Virginia (eighteen months), a secure, close-bonded enclave in an extraordinary household.

On the floor below, Julia's children by her first marriage to Herbert Duckworth were quartered, George, fifteen, Stella, fourteen and Gerald, thirteen. Below that was Leslie and Julia's bedroom, on the first floor the back and principal drawing-rooms, the dining room on the ground floor, with the kitchen and the servants' quarters in the basement. From the attic above the nurseries, Leslie's work-room, the children could hear the rhythmic beat of their father's rocking-chair, functional and elegantly designed in tubular cast-iron with black button-upholstered leather slung like a deckchair, a wooden cross-bar for his feet and another, wider board to hand on which he worked. (This chair, comfortably congruous with the long, bony Stephen frame, was inherited by Adrian who passed it on to his daughters. The chair found a home in the spacious Long Room at the King's Head, looking over the Essex marshes, Adrian and Karin's country home for fifty years, until her death.)

To understand more about the nature of the amalgamated family, the exceptional strains, the strength and confusion of emotions, of unresolved conflicts which came to bear most heavily on Adrian, we must go back and trace something of the lives of the parents, Leslie and Julia Stephen.

Leslie Stephen was born in 1832, at Hyde Park Gate, then named Kensington Gore. His family belonged to the Clapham Sect, a group of like-minded and distinguished friends allied in their

Evangelical religion by their passionate commitment to the cause of Emancipation, the abolition of slavery and freedom for the American negroes. Leslie's forebears were for the most part jurists, civil servants, parliamentarians. With one exception they were not in government; but they used their enormous influence and power as administrators to bear upon Parliament and to penetrate the most influential circles of their day. His father, Sir James Stephen, exchanged his practice at the Bar for a less lucrative post in the Colonial Service in which he rose to become Under-Secretary, as well as doing occasional political journalism. Ten to fifteen years after leaving the Law he was earning £3,000 a year.

In 1814, James Stephen married Catherine Venn who came from a distinguished family of the Clapham Sect. 'Her equable temperament, her singular common sense,' her son Leslie writes, counterbalanced the 'nervous irritability characteristic of the Stephen family', worsened by his father's unlimited capacity for overwork. 'The truth is', as Sir James answered a friend, 'I am not a simple man.' Nor was Leslie himself as he might have admitted. It may have been this which, as we shall see, led him to wish 'simplicity' upon his younger son, Adrian.

Leslie had an affectionate respect for his father. But he loved his mother dearly. He was the third son of a family of five, the youngest and her favourite. She kept a diary in which she recorded his progress: how excitable he was, how active, how he clambered about on chairs and sofas, how wayward he was, passing from fits of violent temper to contrition. He had inherited his father's over-sensitiveness; he could not bear criticism and burst into tears when chided. He shared her passion for poetry. 'She knew by heart all such poetry as was not excluded from the sacred canon. She could repeat Cowper and Wordsworth, Campbell and Scott, and her children learnt "The Mariners of England" and "The Death of Marmion" almost before they could read themselves.'

His mother taught him shorthand (this useful accomplishment was in turn taught to Adrian by his mother); he enjoyed arithmetic. But his mother noted his pallor, his lassitude after only half an hour. Incipient brain fever was diagnosed, poetry forbidden, country air-prescribed. Whereupon Sir James, ever solicitous for his family, removed them all to Brighton where Leslie attended his brother Fitzjames's preparatory school as a day-boy. They moved again to Windsor whence their father, repelled by the brutality and ill-repute of public schools, sent them to Eton as day-boys . No worse fate could have befallen them. They were scorned, tormented and incessantly bullied. Fitzjames afterwards regretted his 'cowardice' in delaying so long before rebelling. Leslie seems to have obliterated the memory of the worst of the bullying though he remembers being rescued more than once by his brother.

Their father thought that Trinity College, which Fitzjames had entered in 1841, would 'overstrain' his younger son and sent Leslie to his own smaller college, Trinity Hall, in 1850, to read for an honours degree in mathematics. For the first time he left behind his family, the constant emphasis on his frailty and uncertain health, and the regime for improving his physique, the Indian clubs and the chest-expander. Like many young people freed from parental over-anxiety, he soon gained confidence and independence of mind and made his own plans for improving his stamina and toughening himself up. He walked prodigious distances; he rowed in the Trinity Hall boat, not well, but he became a first-rate coach.

His shyness at first limited his choice of friends; and for a time he was thought to belong to the 'rowing toughs'. But by his third year, during which he gained first-class honours in the Mathematical tripos, his circle of friends had widened. He had settled into a characteristic turn of speech, vigorous, clear and to the point; and spoke in the Cambridge Debating Union. He was elected to a Fellowship in 1854 for which he had to take Holy Orders. He described himself as 'a vaguely broad churchman'. The Revd Leslie Stephen continued to coach the college boat and was a formidable cross-country runner; he promoted Cambridge athletics, believing that violent, pleasurable exertion was the best way of combating wrong-thinking and wrongdoing and of turning out the manly affectionate young fellows that were his ideal. It is he, Noel Annan claims, not Charles Kingsley, who should be thought of as the founder of muscular Christianity.

Though he took his clerical duties lightly, he thought deeply about the origins of Christianity and examined the tenets of the Church, increasingly repelled by dogma. By 1860 he was steadily reading philosophy; and in 1861 was appointed examiner in the newly created Moral Science tripos. His wide reading in philosophy contributed to loss of faith; by the summer of 1862 he felt himself unable to conduct services in the college chapel. This he was too scrupulous to fudge or conceal, and in 1862 he offered to resign his Fellowship. However, the college was reluctant to lose so good a teacher and he continued to hold his Fellowship until 1864, when he left Cambridge and supported himself by literary and political journalism in London.

Later that year he went to America to make up his own mind about the Civil War. For good reason he supported the North, unlike the majority of his countrymen. During his travels to Washington and New York, and the battlefront, he learnt to appreciate Americans in a way that was rare at home. In New England he met friends of like mind. Three became lifelong friends – Oliver Wendell Holmes, C. E. Norton of Harvard and, closest of all, James Russell Lowell who became Minister to the Court of St James's – and Virginia Stephen's godfather.

From 1865 Leslie lived with his mother and sister in London. 'My life was peaceful and happy.' His work as a journalist made him friends in the literary and political world. With characteristic understatement he wrote to his children: 'I knew various people of more or less reputation' – a list which includes Tennyson, Matthew Arnold, the Brownings, and George Eliot and G. H. Lewes. And he was the model for Vernon Whitford, the idealistic scholar in George Meredith's 1879 novel *The Egoist*.

As Noel Annan notes, Leslie Stephen was uxorious and fortunate in his two marriages. In 1867 he married Harriet Marian (Minny), Thackeray's daughter. He revered women as he reverenced the mountain peaks he climbed in the Swiss Alps: 'I heard one day of [their] approach [to Zermatt] and walked down the valley to meet them. One of my sacred places ever afterwards was a point where the road winds round a little bluff near Täsch. Thence I descried the party approaching on mules . . . and I walked back with them to Zermatt' (*The Mausoleum Book*).

He must have been an arresting figure standing on the bluff waving a wide-brimmed hat, tall, lean, with abundant chestnut hair, small wide-set blue eyes and fine-cut beaky features.

At first they lived in Onslow Gardens, a house owned by Minny and her elder sister Anny. The two were inseparable, and Anny, who by then had begun to make her name as a novelist, lived with them. Her vivacious intelligence was something of a thorn in Leslie's flesh which he bore, on the whole, with resignation. In 1873, they moved to 20 Hyde Park Gate, also part of the Thackeray daughters' property. He had a retaining fee of 50 guineas a year from the editor of the *Saturday Review*. And in 1871 he had been offered the editorship of the *Cornhill Magazine* which brought in £500 a year and enabled him to give up some of his journalism and to 'set about' *The History of English Thought in the Eighteenth Century.* 'I wrote with a certain audacity which I no longer possess . . . I took some things very easily, it seems to me.' From which it may be inferred he was not then the fretful, demanding cantankerous man he had become by the time Virginia and Adrian were born some ten years later; not yet driven by compulsive overwork nor obsessed by largely unfounded money anxieties.

Their domestic life was equally peaceable, though Anny reported to friends that he was 'subject to fits of rage'. After trying 'an independent establishment', Leslie writes, Anny returned and 'took up her abode with us, though it might be said that we took up our abode with her.'

Minny seems to have been equable and affectionate. Leslie thought of her always as a child. Once, in the Zoological Gardens, he noticed the expression on the face of 'one of the darling little foxes' and tenderly remarked, 'You are like my Minny. . . . Its cunning (in the American sense) and apparently amiable little face reminded me of my own dear Minny's expression.' She was intelligent enough to appreciate his literary success and to share his interests and love of the Swiss Alps. They travelled in Europe and America, where he renewed old friendships. Their daughter Laura was born in 1870, a delicate child tenderly watched over by her mother. Minny's health occasionally gave cause for unease, but they went on happily enough 'in unbroken harmony', with frequent visits to the Alps. In 1875 they were *en famille* in Switzerland where Minny, again pregnant, suffered a great deal of discomfort. They returned to Hyde Park Gate. On November 27, late at night, she was taken mortally ill. Earlier that evening Julia Duckworth, who lived next door and was a close friend of them both, looked in and 'found us so happy together that she thought the presence of a desolate widow incongruous, and left us to return to her own solitary hearth'. The next day Minny died, on November 28, Leslie's forty-third birthday. That morning Julia came in. He remembers 'how tenderly she kissed me'.

Julia Prinsep Jackson had been born in India in 1846. Her mother, Maria (*née* Pattle) brought her to England in 1848. At first they lived in Hendon, then in Well Walk, Hampstead, settling eventually in Kent, in a house called Saxonbury. Here Dr Jackson, 'a worthy and eminently respectable person' – so Leslie Stephen, his son-in-law, describes him – joined them on his retirement.

Maria Jackson was one of the seven Pattle sisters renowned for their beauty in an Anglo-Indian family of some distinction and occasional eccentricity. Maria's sister Sara had married Thoby Prinsep, a retired Anglo-Indian administrator. He and Sara lived in Little Holland House, an agreeable, large, rambling house on the edge of London, in what is now Melbury Road. Their informal hospitality attracted painters, writers and statesmen such as Tennyson, Thackeray, Meredith, Gladstone and Disraeli. George Frederic Watts came for a long visit and stayed on indefinitely, with his studios at the top of the house. Sara and Thoby Prinsep welcomed the established and succoured the unfortunate – Sara, it was claimed, saved the young Burne-Jones's life. Julia's two elder sisters, Adeline and Mary, were already there, cousins came and went, so Mrs Jackson and Julia were a natural addition to the extended family.

Thus she virtually grew up in a lively, stimulating environment. For her own father, so long absent during her formative years, she felt dutiful affection; but she adored her uncle Thoby, her father-figure. She remained close to her mother during her lifetime and, after her sisters' early marriages, became her favourite daughter.

Virginia remembered her mother,[3] as seen in a lost photograph, stepping out on to the lawn one summer's afternoon about 1860; and we can imagine her in 'a striped silk dress buttoned at the neck with a flowing skirt' moving among her friends in the gardens of Little Holland House, the croquet lawn, the shrubberies, the tea-tables, dispensing strawberries, sugar and cream, bending her lovely head to listen and respond, well-bred, charming, unaffected, amused, altogether lovable.

Her elders adored her. She was drawn and painted by George Frederic Watts; Edward Burne-Jones made her his model for his picture of the Annunciation; her aunt, Julia Cameron, photographed her, Henry Taylor wrote a poem about her when they met at Tennyson's house in the Isle of Wight – he had gone there to meet Garibaldi. Holman Hunt and Woolner, the sculptor, both asked for her hand in marriage.

In 1862, when Julia was sixteen, she went with her mother to Venice where her sister Mary and Herbert Fisher were on their honeymoon. He had been taken ill; and in the admirable way that Victorians undertook long and wearisome journeys abroad, mother and daughter immediately set out to support bride and groom. Here Julia met Herbert Duckworth, a friend of Herbert Fisher's. There is no vulgar suggestion of 'love at first sight' in Leslie Stephen's account in *The Mausoleum Book*. But the two met again at

[3] *Moments of Being*

intervals, generally abroad, where Mrs Jackson travelled in search of cures for her rheumatism.

They became engaged in February 1867, and were married from Saxonbury on May 4, when he was thirty-four, she just twenty-one. As a rising barrister he had joined the Northern Circuit and she accompanied him everywhere; the shortest separation threw her into a state of agitation. But their idyllic marriage was cut short after fewer than four years by his sudden death in September 1870, leaving her with two children, George and Stella; Gerald was born ten days after his father's death.

Writing after her death, Leslie Stephen thought that she had a concept of marriage unusual at the time. She believed that a woman ought either to refuse a man unconditionally or to accept him unreservedly. He goes on to write that there was something alarming in the spectacle of a pure-minded young woman, ignorant of the fullest meaning of marriage, surrendering herself so utterly. But Mr Duckworth was an honourable and suitable man, worthy, Leslie had to admit, of her devotion. Whether any man could have responded on her exalted plane we shall never know; he had only to accept, and to fulfil their passion on a human scale. She enshrined her ideal of marriage in their short, perfect union; and preserved the memory till her death.

Her life, she wrote, 'seemed a shipwreck'. But her mother and her children needed her. 'I knew I had to live on and on, and the only thing to be done was to be as cheerful as I could and do as much as I could and think as little as I could. And so I got deadened.' If she had been able to be more true to herself, had allowed herself to break down, she believed she could have 'got more real life out of the wreck'.

She found a way of living on through consoling the bereaved and tending the sick, a duty which might have led to a lifelong vocation: she learnt the skills of nursing. Her book, *Notes From Sick Rooms*, privately printed in 1883 and reissued in 1980, written with humour and acumen, shows how her sensitivity to suffering was combined with practical understanding of her patients' needs. She knew how even the smallest adjustments could relieve discomfort. She learnt the techniques of preparing and offering food, of alleviating nausea, of giving an enema, of laying out the dead.

She had been diffident in approaching Leslie fancying that she 'bored' him. But his bereavement brought them closer. Another bond was her loss of religious faith after her husband's death; she became an agnostic. She soon felt able to chide Leslie on various points, on his behaviour to Anny whose want of sense about money matters drove him to distraction. 'Julia spoke to me more to the purpose about my want of temper. I took a turn with her in Kensington Gardens, when I had the sense to confess my shortcomings. She, I could see, was pleased at my willingness to listen to reason, and we became, I think, better friends from that day.' There were difficulties too about Laura's nurse, Louise, whom he trusted too implicitly.

Most importantly, there was the affair between Anny and Richmond Ritchie, a man much younger than herself. He was at the house almost every day; and Leslie, outraged, found them kissing in the drawing-room. Julia's good sense was invaluable. He hated the match, she suggested to him, partly because 'all men are jealous and I might feel I was being put at a lower level in Anny's affections. . . . I hated it because men at least always hate a marriage between a young man and an older woman.' As Julia had foretold, the marriage proved very happy.

It may be seen from these frank exchanges and constant meetings that he had begun to realise the 'enormous value of her friendship and to depend more and more on her judgement', specially when his household was broken up by Anny's leaving. Yet she still found him alarming, still feared that she bored him, an uncertainty which continued till he returned from his first winter expedition to the Alps in 1877. 'She had however discovered that something less repulsive was concealed by my alarming outside.' As for him, he was walking into town one day past Knightsbridge barracks when it came upon him as a flash of revelation: 'I am in love with Julia!'

He wrote a note declaring his love, saying that he knew she did not reciprocate his feeling, and that marriage between them was out of the question. He was writing, he said – and he handed her the note as she left after a dinner party at his house – because he could not help himself; and because if he had to cease seeing her without explanation the break would be inexplicable, unforgivable. She took the note with 'a little glance of surprise'. Almost at once he heard a knock at the door. 'My darling had read the letter and returned on the impulse of the moment.' She patted his shoulder 'tenderly and caressingly' and told him he had rightly divined her feelings. Their marriage, she said, was out of the question. They were to continue 'on the terms of closest friendship but never upon closer terms'.

During that year they saw one another constantly. When they

were separated they wrote to one another daily, sometimes oftener. Extracts printed in *The Mausoleum Book* show how seriously she thought about their friendship, how candidly she expressed her views. Leslie indicates the multiplicity of her reasons for wanting to keep matters between them as they had been; but without the letters, which on his showing became on both sides more intimate, more lover-like, we cannot know in full what led her in the end to surrender.

On 5 January, 1878, 'I went in to sit with her one evening. We talked the matter over once more and I rose to go. . . . Suddenly she looked up and said, "I will be your wife and will do my best to be a good wife to you!" "All doubts vanished like a dream," she writes to me from Freshwater. "My darling one, I feel most commonplace and quiet. The only thing I can't quite believe is that we are not married."'

They were married at St Mary's Church, Kensington, on March 26, 1878.

Leslie and Laura moved from 20 to 22 Hyde Park Gate, her house. Soon, to accommodate their growing family, two storeys were added. In 1879 Vanessa was born, followed by Julian Thoby, 1880, Adeline Virginia, 1882, and Adrian Leslie, 1883. (The last two were unplanned, rudimentary birth control having failed them.) By the age of forty-two she had borne seven children, besides having taken on Laura, who before long showed signs of insanity. (She was eventually put in the care of a doctor who specialised in mental disorders.) Whatever the Duckworth children felt about the change in their lives they must have needed extra thought and attention. Above all she had taken on a husband whose grief and the sense of being abandoned when Minny died increased his nervous irritability and shortened his temper – witness the talks and the gentle chiding in Kensington Gardens before their marriage.

Most parents, by the time their family is completed, have shaken down into some degree of habitual conjugality, at worst a tacit acceptance of mutual dissatisfaction, at best a union of affectionate understanding, providing a stable framework such as Leslie Stephen's own family. But he and Julia had had no time to settle. He revered her; she was, he said, 'his saint'. She had her own preoccupations; her ideal husband, her first marriage, kept a place in her heart.

In 1883, the year of Adrian's birth, Leslie, aged fifty-one, embarked on the work on which (as he foresaw to his regret) his reputation rests: he became the creator and first editor of the *Dictionary of National Biography.* This laborious and uncongenial task, involving endless discussions with contributors, printers, etc, continued till, in 1891, he gave it up. He wrote many of the best contributions himself. It had taxed his energy almost to breaking-point and greatly increased his irascibility.

Julia schooled herself to manage him, to meet his excessive demands and shield the children from his worst tempers. But her effort was not without its effect on her health and inner strength. Adrian, his sister Virginia wrote, 'was squeezed in the womb' by the *Dictionary.*

We cannot doubt that these two remarkable people, Leslie and Julia Stephen, loved one another deeply; but they were not settled in their relationship. Children are unconsciously aware of the inner feelings of those closest to them. And Adrian had the misfortune, in this respect at least, to be her favourite.

3

EARLY DAYS

For a time nursery life kept up its daily rhythm 'with great simplicity and regularity', as Virginia Woolf describes it. 'It seems to divide itself into two large spaces, not crowded with events but in some way more exquisitely natural than any that follows; for our duties were very plain and our pleasures absolutely appropriate. . . . One space was spent in the drawing-room and nursery, and the other in Kensington Gardens. There were a number of little warfares, and some times Vanessa and Thoby fought with us and some times they were our friends. . . . The Others (the Duckworth children) were not brothers and sisters but beings possessed of knives or enviable gifts for running and carving.' (*Moments of Being*, Virginia Woolf)

At first Vanessa was attached to Thoby, fourteen months younger than herself, though she kept a motherly eye on the two younger ones. Thoby, Virginia wrote, was her special care. Before long, however, she and Virginia came together in a close companionship that lasted all their lives.

When they were grown up, Virginia, distressed by Adrian's unhappiness, felt guilty at her early desertion, believing she should not have tacked on to the others and left him on his own. She need not have felt guilty; his difficulties were attributable to other causes.

Adrian was his mother's favourite, her 'Benjamin', as Leslie Stephen wrote after her death. She adored him, called him 'her joy'; she kept his photograph in the drawing-room where she could always see it, and another beside her bed. Inevitably this must have caused jealousy among the others, not to speak of her possessive husband.

Leslie Stephen had a strange view of his younger son, indicative of his own mixed feelings: 'Adrian is an attractive simple little fellow but oddly dreamy and apt to take an interest in things that are impracticable.' (That letter to his friend, Charles Eliot Norton, was not, as might be supposed, written when Adrian was an infant, but when he was eleven-and-a-half, soon after his mother's death.) Adrian was never simple. Nor was he dreamy; intent, rather, on the matter in hand. Children have moth-like antennae; they sense what their parents want of them and early on adopt an image which is often far from their innermost thoughts and unconscious feelings. They expected him to be dreamy, unpractical – and so he outwardly remained. Inwardly he had a rebellious streak, the making of a rebel. He had been named, his father wrote, after Adrian Scrope,[4] 'a fine old regicide from whom the Stephens claimed descent – how I don't know'.

When did Julia make time to be with her children? Virginia writes:

> Can I ever remember being alone with her for more than a few minutes? She was always being interrupted. . . . She was the most prompt, practical and vivid of human beings. . . . Most often her service, when it was not purely practical, lay in simply helping people in the light of her judgment and experience to see what they really meant or felt. . . . All her gifts had something swift, decisive, witty even, in their nature; so that there could be no question of dulness or drudgery in her daily work, however lugubrious it seemed of itself. She was sensitive by temperament and impatient of stupidity; and while she was there the whole of that interminable and incongruous procession which is the life of a large family, went merrily.

Julia's mother was her constant care; she wrote almost daily to Mrs Jackson, ready to go to her when she was ill; she had her commitment to the sick, the poor; and there were friends and relatives to be nursed, sometimes at distances which took her away from home. As to daily occupations, there was her complex household to run – she was an exacting mistress, though sympathetic to genuine distress.

[4] Adrian Scrope, 1601–60 Raised troop of horse for the Parliament army. Major inf Regt of Horse 1646. When Army and Parliament quarrelled he took part of the soldiers. Appointed one of the King's judges. Signed the death warrant. Tried as regicide and executed at Charing Cross 1660. Described when in prison and on the gallows as 'a comely, ancient gentleman'.

She taught her children Latin, history and French herself, believing she could do it better than a governess. Their father attempted to teach them mathematics, a trial to them all!

In the afternoons there might be social calls to pay, accompanied by her eldest daughter, Stella. Vanessa and Virginia learnt in their turn by example the social graces proper to well-brought-up Victorian girls. More importantly there were her duties as the wife of a distinguished husband, formal engagements, dinners at home. Always her first care was for him, calming his anxieties, bearing the brunt of his irascibility, both of them bowed under the terrible *Dictionary*. At her tea-table there might be eminent friends, writers, statesmen; and innumerable cousins, Stephens, Prinseps, Vaughans, Fishers; elderly bores into whom she sparked life; young men – she was always interested in them and was something of a matchmaker. The younger children might be brought down from the nursery.

As to Adrian's early life almost all is conjecture. But we know enough about his mother to be reasonably sure that from babyhood she gave him confidence; though he might fret when she was absent, he soon learnt that she would always return. Later, secure in their close relationship, though he shared in her happiness 'tinged with sadness,'[5] his latent sense of her suppressed emotional conflict could have been a responsibility that gave him the thoughtful look evident in all but one of the family photographs.

The best time for them all was when they decamped for the summer to St Ives on the north coast of Cornwall. In 1881 Leslie Stephen, walking from Penzance to the little fishing-port on the westernmost promontory of England, found Talland House, a sizeable roomy house in a large garden high above the town with a sweeping view over Carbis Bay. He saw that it would make a holiday house for the family and, in spite of his obsession about money, weighed up in his methodical way the cost and the logistics of transporting his family some three hundred miles to 'the toenail of England', and leased the house from the Great Western Railway. The place was ideal and for thirteen summers the family enjoyed a brief idyllic happiness.

In Cornwall underlying tensions were relaxed. The *Dictionary* lessened its hold on their father, who played lightheartedly with his children. A friend remembers him drawing his naked children through his legs into the waves. When they were old enough he took them on walks round the peninsula or over the moors. He

[5] *Moments of Being*, Virginia Woolf

taught them the names and families of plants and encouraged their bug-hunting and their collections of moths and butterflies.

Julia's bright spirit was at the heart of their summers at St Ives. Forever occupied, as in London, with the same cares, her household to run, lessons as usual, and with the added pleasurable distraction of friends, not forgetting visits to the town, a basket in her arm, to comfort the sick and the needy, she yet found time, more time than at home, to be with her children. She would go with the younger ones under the railway tunnel that led to the shore and there spend the day while Leslie took the older contingent on long walks. She sat there on the beach in quiet content, with Laura her stepdaughter, and the dog, Shag.

There was time, always, to take her husband's arm and lead him away to some quiet part of the garden to calm his rages; to recover for both their abiding love for each other.

Adrian could have been three-and-a-half or so when he first became aware of the joys of anticipation, beginning with the journey across London to Paddington, a royal progress with the elders in at least two four-wheelers followed by servants, nurses and children in cabs piled high with all the paraphernalia needed for a three-month exodus. If spirits flagged during the long train journey, they revived as the train drew into St Erth's where they changed on to the branch line for St Ives. At last Adrian, lifted down by his father, holding his mother's hand, drew in his first breath of soft, salty Cornish air. Then up the drive to Talland House, standing on the terrace surveying the twilit bay, the lights of the town, the lighthouse whose beam swept all night over sleeping children at the top of the high, spare house open to the winds and the sound of the sea. 'After the months in London, to go away to Cornwall; to have our own house, our own garden; to have the Bay; the sea; the moors . . . to hear the waves breaking that first night behind the yellow blind.'

Grown-ups came to stay but the children never asked friends of their own. '"Us four" were completely self-sufficient.' It is on the cricket lawn that Adrian's first surviving photograph was taken. He is batting, Virginia properly alert, the wicket-keeper. (Cricket was taken seriously: the Stephens were coached by their half-brother George who had played for Eton. He bowled to them in the basement passage at Hyde Park Gate.) Here Adrian is not serious; that round, merry face is all impish delight. He is said to be three in the photograph – three-and-three-quarters – so Virginia would be five-and-a-half; she looks older. Beside her Adrian looks small, as indeed he was, specially compared with his tall family, until, in his early teens, he grew and overtopped them all. For years he believed he was a dwarf.

In her novel, *To The Lighthouse*, on the first page Virginia describes her brother Adrian:

> 'Yes, of course, if it's fine to-morrow,' said Mrs Ramsay. 'But you'll have to be up with the lark,' she added.
>
> To her son these words conveyed an extraordinary joy, as if it were settled the expedition were bound to take place, and the wonder to which he had looked forward, for years and years it seemed, was, after a night's darkness and a day's sail, within touch. Since he belonged, even at the age of six, to that great clan which cannot keep this feeling separate from that, but must let future prospects, with their joys and sorrows, cloud what is actually at hand, since to such people even in earliest childhood any turn in the wheel of sensation has the power to crystallise and transfix the moment upon which its gloom or radiance rests, James Ramsay, sitting on the floor cutting out pictures from the illustrated catalogue of the Army and Navy Stores, endowed the picture of a refrigerator as his mother spoke with heavenly bliss. It was fringed with joy. The wheelbarrow, the lawnmower, the sound of poplar trees, leaves whitening before rain, rooks cawing, brooms knocking, dresses rustling – all these were so coloured and distinguished in his mind that he had already his private code, his secret language, though he appeared the image of stark and uncompromising severity, with his high forehead and his fierce blue eyes, impeccably candid and pure, frowning slightly at the sight of human frailty, so that his mother, watching him guide his scissors neatly round the refrigerator, imagined him all red and ermine on the Bench or directing a stern and momentous enterprise in some crisis of public affairs.

4

JULIA'S DEATH

The year 1891 was remarkable for at least two events. Firstly, Leslie Stephen gave up his editorship of the *Dictionary of National Biography*, to the relief of his wife and children. Julia had become increasingly anxious about its effects on his health; he had already had to rest for three months after a 'seizure'. Secondly, the *Hyde Park Gate News* began publication, written and edited by Vanessa and Virginia. It appeared regularly every Monday throughout 1891 and 1892 and, though two years are missing, survived until May 1895 and their mother's death. There is uncertainty as to who wrote what; from a scholarly comparison of their handwriting it would seem that the entries are fairly well divided.

The *Hyde Park Gate News*, written tongue-in-cheek in the convention of a 'quality' newspaper gossip column, gives an immediate day-to-day account of family life. And a lively, talented family they were, remarkably unconstrained compared with the rigid standards of the time. Their father, for all his cantankerousness was, on his own terms, very much a part of family life. He took them on his own favourite treat, the Zoological Gardens. In Cornwall he played with them when they were young, and he took them on excursions when they were old enough, botanising and infusing them with his own interests. His participation in their lives was brought about by his wife, but the price she paid unstintingly for the management of this almost unmanageable man was her increasing exhaustion and debility. Her children led the life she planned for them for as long as she lived.

And Adrian was very much part of this life. He was ribbed, squashed and laughed at by his sisters, and like others who are the youngest in a family he strove to be different, to excel in his own way, at once imitative and idiosyncratic; for instance, he started rival newspapers which were bound to fail and were mercilessly mocked by his siblings. But his secure place in their affections, in the fabric of their young lives, is clear from the pages of the *Hyde Park Gate News.*

In the issue of December 7, 1891, we learn that Mr Leslie Stephen on retiring from the editorship of the *DNB* was given a pair of silver candlesticks and a snuffer tray. On Monday, December 21, 1891, there was a dancing class for the Stephens 'including Master Adrian Stephen'. On May 30, 1892 Stella's and Vanessa's joint birthday was celebrated by Mrs Stephen taking them with Virginia 'in a suffocating carriage' to watch Thoby's school play cricket.

At the foot of one number is a diagram captioned 'NODES by Our Astronomer'. This is evidently by Adrian since, according to the *Hyde Park Gate News*, 'Master Adrian Stephen' was the only member of the family who shared their mother's interest in astronomy. 'Let us suppose', writes Our Astronomer, 'that the circles in the following picture are planets forming nodes.' A clearly drawn diagram follows: 'The dotted line EF is called the line of the nodes because it passes through the edges of the planets which cut each other or are on a level with each other.' This scientific contribution – he was not yet nine years old – affords an early specimen of a style that he retained in later life: concise, accurate and informative rather than imaginative.

September 8 was Thoby's birthday and the entry of that week shows the source of the opening chapter of *To The Lighthouse.*

> On Saturday morning Master Hilary Hunt and Master Basil Smith came up to Talland House and asked Master Thoby and Miss Virginia Stephen to accompany them to the lighthouse as Freeman the boatman said that there was a perfect tide and wind for going there. Master Adrian Stephen was much disappointed at not being allowed to go.

Late in October the *News* records the family's return to London. Adrian's ninth birthday (October 27) was celebrated with a party, presents and crackers. Mr Burne-Jones came to tea and 'acts as a sort of moving spirit to everything'. On Saturday, October 28, Leslie, Virginia and Adrian visited the school to see Thoby play football against the Old Etonians. Much to their father's disgust they took bugs, chrysalides and butterflies to the dormitory and arranged the butterflies on Thoby's bedside locker, spilling most of the bran they had been packed in. They saw where the boys' pets were kept, and fondled the Himalayan rabbits.

The November 21 issue records that Leslie Stephen was made President of the London Library, an honourable position previously held by Carlyle, Tennyson and other distinguished men. 'The greater part of Mrs Stephen's joy lies in the fact that Mr Gladstone is only Vice-President. She is not at all of a "crowy" nature but we can forgive any woman for triumphing when her husband gets above Mr Gladstone.'

In January 1892 Adrian had joined Thoby at Evelyn's. 'The baby (but alas! he is no longer one) has returned to Evelyn's. He departed . . . last Thursday at 5.30 p.m. taking with him 50 oranges.'

Evelyn's School, at Colham Green near Hillingdon, Middlesex, was founded in 1872 by G. T. Worsley, and only closed in 1931. It was soundly based educationally; and Mr and Mrs Worsley between them provided a civilised, relaxed atmosphere that was remarkably humane for the times. If, as Adrian wrote, there were sixty-three boys, the staff was large and there seem to have been no harsh or second-rate masters. George and Gerald Duckworth had been there; and Leslie Stephen deserves credit for his two sons following them. Like his father before him, he cared for their well-being, and in the Evangelical tradition valued the connection between school and home.

Adrian, who entered Evelyn's shortly after his ninth birthday, settled into what was already a familiar environment. He wrote to his mother every Sunday and she supplied him with stamped postcards to get a mid-weekly report, often on his health.

His letters for the year 1894 and the first third of 1895 have survived. They are, it must be said, more varied, more amusing and better written than Thoby's which give the impression of a cheerful, athletic, and generally popular boy. Adrian remains more in touch with his family than is common when children go away to school; he asks about the girls, about the dog, Shag, and the cat: 'Have you caught many mice recently?' A cryptic entry: 'Did Nessa and Stella enjoy their trip to Constantinople?' (There is no record of this unlikely excursion.)

He generally prefaces his letters by a comment on his place in form: 'February 21 1894. I came out top this week. Mr Knowles was very surprised when I told him I had done the whole of Rust,[6] and a little Greek and he said he thought I should get into the fifth next term. Good bye your loving Adrian.'

[6] Rust, a Latin grammar or primer

Adrian is always losing things or leaving them behind, books, pencil-cases, toothbrushes and sponges. ('The water is always hot. We have baths four times a week.') He confidently expects them to be replaced or sent on. His interest in astronomy is kept up. 'There is a fine sun-spot,' he writes to his mother, 'but you must look at it through smoke.'

There is a last postcard postmarked February 15, 1895: 'Dear Mother, My name is down for a chess tournament. I am 3d this week . . . the measles have not spread. I have just got your letter. Good bye your loving Adrian.' (He was in bed with measles.)

In February, 1895, during very severe weather, their mother was confined to bed with influenza. After a fortnight, though still very weak, she was allowed to sit up in Stella's bedroom. On March 11, we learn from the *Hyde Park Gate News*, she came downstairs and lay on the sofa with strict instructions not to move which she ignored, going about, answering letters and superintending the household. She announced her intention of going to see Adrian, still at school with measles; but the weather was so stormy even she had to give up the attempt. On March 8 Adrian was brought home. Their mother was improving and 'insists on getting up for breakfast'. After the April holidays Adrian returned to school.

It seemed that Julia had recovered. But two months later she suffered a relapse; and on May 11, with shocking suddenness, she died.

Her death was an appalling loss for the whole family. But on Adrian its effect can hardly be imagined. Thoby had been telegraphed; he was met at Paddington by George, Vanessa and Virginia. Who told Adrian? Who met him at Paddington? He must have been with them all when they were taken in to her deathbed by Stella. But his presence then, and later, is a blank, as though he had become wraithlike. Perhaps that was what he felt himself to be.

5

COPING WITH BEREAVEMENT

Leslie Stephen's massive egocentricity found full force at his wife's death. His noisy grief left no room for consideration of his children. It was George who woke Vanessa and Virginia in the early morning, Stella who brought them down in their dressing-gowns, Stella who took them in to see Julia, still warm. They huddled outside her room until Leslie came out, brushing aside Virginia's instinctive gesture, her hand stretched out to comfort him.

There followed the trappings of Victorian mourning, black clothes, black-edged writing paper, drawn blinds darkening the already dark house; worse, the constant, over-profuse tearful intrusion of relatives and friends which went on for months, inhibiting the children's true, private mourning.

As for Adrian's part in all this, the obsequies, the long drive to Highgate Cemetery, one can only hope that he passed through it with a mercifully blank mind.

Stella, never Julia's favourite, but adoring her, living in her shadow, attempted to take her place. She did her best to console her half-sisters and brothers with gestures of affection and care for their daily comfort. And Adrian began, tentatively, to transfer his dependence on to her. But the family had never had a natural, intimate relationship with the Duckworths and Stella's inability to share her grief with them was disheartening. They might come upon her in tears; but to 'their infinite confusion' she would hide them instantly and make some trivial remark. Worse, she had to meet the daily onset of her stepfather's frenzied ill-temper and outrageous demands.

On the whole the boys returning to school had the easiest part. At least the Worsleys' reasonable sympathy and the familiar round of school life could be counted on to get Adrian through from day to day.

Meanwhile his father found a way of channelling his anguish. On May 25 he began to write a memoir intended for his children into which he poured 'the emotional power of an intricate, fascinating and usually hidden personality'.[7]

He could be frank and objective about what he felt himself and often percipient about the feelings of others. But these qualities were frequently overlaid by sentimentality and mawkish unconvincing professions of love for his children. One passage (on p. 85) is worth quoting exemplifying in full the foregoing aspects of Leslie Stephen's personality; and showing the complexity of his feelings about Adrian, a blindness to his own hostility towards the child. On the one hand he shows a keenly perceptive understanding of his wife's love for their son. In contrast there is the unconscious malice, the belittlement of *'my dear little Adrian, as the youngest of you, will probably have the least distinct impression of his mother'* (my italics). Small wonder that Adrian's early fear and hatred hardened into cold withdrawal.

> I shall just add one thing. I can not say, nor, I am sure, could she have said which of her children she loved best. Rather it was plain that she loved them all equally or that her love for any one of you became most obvious as that one happened to need it most. But, if I may say so, you must all have noticed that though a mother's love for two children may be equal, the love for one has sometimes a peculiar tenderness, caused perhaps by special need or simply from special affinity of character. Now my dear little Adrian, as the youngest of you, will probably have the least distinct impression of his mother. To him, therefore, I shall say that she had a very marked and tender sentiment about her 'Benjamin'. There was something, I cannot define it, which gave a pathetic turn to her emotions where he was concerned. I have been much struck by a likeness, which Stella pointed out to me, between Adrian and the beautiful drawing of his mother by Watts at an early age. Perhaps this indicates some special affinity of temperament, or possibly it was that Adrian showed a special clinging to her. Anyhow, he touched a very soft place in her tender heart. She always called him her 'joy' – or by way of a quaint diminutive 'joydé'. His photographs by Henry Cameron were by her bedside and placed so that her eyes could rest upon them from her habitual seat in the drawing-

[7] *The Mausoleum Book*, Introduction by Alan Bell, OUP.

room. To hear her even pronounce his name was delightful.[8]

An additional reason for Leslie Stephen's prejudice may have been a real or fancied resemblance to himself as a boy. He, too, had had a close relationship with his mother, had had a 'skin too few', had been prone to tears and had deemed himself a weakling; but at least he had laboured to toughen himself up and overcome his childhood failings. Adrian made no effort in that direction. His depressed aloofness must have been a thorn in the side of a forlorn parent striving to be a 'good' father, needing the reassurance of the children's positive response.

Thoby had always been his favourite, promising to fulfil his ideal of what a boy should be. Eighty-eight of Leslie's letters to Thoby, from 1888 to 1903, exist. They show him at his best, often amused and amusing, natural, unaffectedly fond; he addresses Thoby as 'my beloved', or 'my darling Thoby', closing with, 'Goodbye, my darling boy, your loving father'.

During those early years following their mother's death everyone must have looked forward to Thoby's return from school, sharing their sorrow but bringing comfort with his sturdy outlook on life. In 1895, that first long, hot summer without their mother, they went to Freshwater in the Isle of Wight. (Gerald being dispatched to sell the lease of Talland House.) Virginia, on the verge of her first breakdown, remembers it as the most miserable time of all. Freshwater, she wrote, was stuffy, steamy, the vegetation over-luxuriant. But she also recalls how, unexpectedly, 'the first impulse to set us free' came from their father. 'On a walk perhaps he would suddenly brush aside all our curiously conventional relationships and allow us for a minute an inspiriting vision of free life, bathed in an impersonal light. There were a number of things to be learnt, books to be read, and success and happiness were to be attained there without disloyalty. Indeed it seemed possible at these moments, to continue the old life but in a more significant way, using as he told us, our sorrow to quicken the feeling that remained.'

The following summer of 1896 was marked by an important event, Stella's engagement to Jack Waller Hills. The family were staying at Hindhead House, Haslemere, Surrey, and he bicycled over to renew his suit. She had twice refused him, but his quiet persistence was not to be deflected. He was an old friend of the family, approved of by Julia, but not by Leslie, who on this occasion

[8] Ibid.

behaved with his customary crustiness, worsened by a sense of betrayal, of being deprived of someone so necessary to his comfort. That night Stella and Jack went out to the wooded garden and did not return till late. There was an air of crisis, drama, 'fatality almost'. The children were sent up to bed and sat in Adrian's room while their father paced up and down the terrace. At last Stella came up 'blushing the loveliest rose colour, and told us – how she was very happy'. Her stepfather followed, and spoke sharply to Adrian who, perhaps feeling that another calamity had occurred and that he was to suffer a further loss, burst into tears. He should be happy, his father cried, they should all be happy at Stella's happiness – but then lamented that the blow was irreparable.

He insisted on a long engagement, and Stella was still at home that September when Adrian entered Westminster School as a day-boy. She mothered him, retrieved books, gloves, boots, and waved him away at the gate.

Adrian's dependence on Stella only lasted for a year. She was married in 1897; and died three months later from peritonitis associated with pregnancy. It was Vanessa's turn to take on her father, to bear his cruel onslaughts over the weekly household bills. The unpleasant truth is that this frenetic behaviour was directed at women, first, presumably, Julia, then Stella, now Vanessa. In fact there was never any realistic need for anxiety about money. He was said to be alarmed if he had less than £1,000 in his current account. He suffered from what a psychoanalyst[9] has termed 'hypochondriasis of the pocket', meaning that he had given so much to his family he felt drained, emptied.

Virginia remembers how she and Vanessa followed Stella's example, presiding over the breakfast table, waving Adrian away from the gate – he was the first to go, then Jack Hills, then Gerald, lastly George, usually in a hansom cab. And how they all came home to the tea-table, 'Adrian from Westminster; Jack from Clifford's Inn Fields, Gerald from Dent's [the publishers], George from the Post Office or the Treasury, back to the focus, the tea-table where Nessa and I presided'.[10] So the girls kept life going in 'the great echoing shell of a house', but each was preoccupied, seizing what leisure remained to do her own work, Vanessa at an art school, Virginia at her classical studies – and she was beginning to write. They were often absent, visiting friends, as were George and Gerald. Adrian must have frequently come home to an empty

9 Leslie Sohn

10 From *Moments of Being*

house or, worse still, to an evening alone with his father. There is pathos in a photograph taken during their summer holidays in 1897 at Painswick. One cannot but feel sympathy for them both, the elderly father making a tentative gesture as though to put his arm round Adrian's shoulder, and the bleak look on Adrian's face, staring ahead, dressed ready to return to school.

Leslie's hopes rested on Thoby, for whom his love grew into an obsession. In his diary he records his progress at school, his measles, his mumps, more alarmingly his two bouts of pneumonia, and his progress at work. There is scant mention of Adrian except his entry to Westminster in 1896, and another following in 1897: 'Adrian seems to be getting acclimatized at Westminster.' And in the same entry, 'Thoby is doing well at Clifton, having waked up from some slackness due to rapid growth.'

In November 1897 Thoby got an exhibition at Trinity – 'The best piece of news I have had for some time.'

Not all Adrian's holidays can have left him so depressed as the Painswick summer. In 1898 Leslie took the family to the Manor House, Ringwood, on the verge of the New Forest. He enjoyed it and hoped his family, and the friends they invited, did so too. One may reasonably surmise that the young Stephens, schooled in London by their riding-master, learned there to ride in earnest, cantering down grassy rides between massive, ancient trees, glimpsing antlered deer, or the rare sight of a roe and her pricket crossing a ride in the green twilight. And there were long gallops across open heathland on higher ground.

For many years riding was Adrian's favourite exercise. He and Thoby rode at Cambridge and hunted when they could afford it; and their horsemanship was put through an exacting test during their expedition to Montenegro and Greece in 1906.

The Stephens returned to the New Forest in the summer of 1900, this time to Frithan House, Lyndhurst; and again in 1901. In 1902 Thoby, still at Cambridge, invited his friend Lytton Strachey to visit them, and Lytton writes to Leonard Woolf, 'What is strange is the old man – older than he really is – among so young a family. He is well kept in check by them, and they are well bustled by him. They know each other very well, I think.' And so they did, towards the end of Leslie's life. They could laugh at his growing eccentricities, and receive only mild reproof. There is a well-known story of Adrian's mimicry of their deaf father's voice unheard by him at the dinner table. But when Adrian tried it in a cab the acoustics relayed the sound like an ear-trumpet. Even then Leslie, much distressed, only lamented, 'Oh, my boy, my boy.'

1901 was a memorable year for Adrian. In September Leslie arranged for him to board at 'Tanner's House'. 'Accounts of his school progress were unsatisfactory and I hope that he may have a better chance there. His great growth – over 6ft 2in – has tried him.' (Adrian had grown six inches in one year and was to attain 6ft 5in.)[11]

From then on his chances did indeed improve. He had the good fortune to be 'up-Grant's' under a remarkable housemaster, Ralph Tanner. Adrian, as his letters to his mother show, had been a bright, even a reasonably ambitious boy, and with Ralph Tanner he found an incentive to recover his powers. He began to take part in house activities. The *Grantite Review* records that he joined the Literary Society in 1901; and he played chess: 'There has been a house chess tournament of which (*sic*) ALS is the moving spirit.' In the Literary Society play-reading of *The Merchant of Venice*, 'Stephen as Salanio and H. Logan as Salarino gave some indication of what they were to do in the future.'

'In The *School for Scandal* Stephen's reading of Sir Oliver and Mrs Candour was one of the features of a most successful reading.'

On October 10 the House debated the motion 'That this House approves of vaccination.' Mr A. L. Stephen and Mr Ashley, in opposing the motion, referred to the German Army and the Italian Army, 'quoting various doubtful statistics'.

In 1902 Adrian got his 3rd eleven football colours. In the same term he got into the semi-finals of the chess tournament. He played cricket in season.

These entries, sparse though they are, show characteristics that were to become important: Adrian wanted to be an actor; and his career as a barrister, had he pursued it wholeheartedly, would have been a way of expressing his histrionic talent.

He passed the entrance examination for Trinity at Easter 1902, and went up in October.

[11] Information Ann Synge.

6

CAMBRIDGE

When Adrian went up to Trinity Thoby returned with him for a fourth year. He had failed to get the first-class degree in Classics which would have entitled him to go on to an academic career. His father, much disappointed, wrote in June that Thoby had 'taken it bravely' and was 'off to Freiburg to cram German'. His return to Cambridge was, his father believed, 'to cram for the Civil Service exam', a plan which seems to have changed. For in 1905, Thoby wrote to Leonard Woolf that he was in chambers studying law.

Thoby made a strong, lasting impression on all who knew him. He had gone up to Cambridge in 1899 with a group of undergraduates, among them Lytton Strachey, Leonard Woolf, Clive Bell and Saxon Sydney-Turner. One and all they acclaimed Thoby, took him for their own, seem from a distance to have closed round him in a charmed circle. Much has been preserved through their memories, the more sharply defined for being crowded into the few years before his early death. Leonard Woolf wrote of his friend:

> He gave one an impression of physical magnificence. He was six foot two, broad-shouldered and somewhat heavily made. He had many of the characteristic qualities of the males of his family, of his father Leslie Stephen, his uncle James Fitzjames Stephen and his cousin J. K. Stephen. But what everyone who knew him remembers most vividly in him was his extraordinary charm. He had greater personal charm than anyone I have ever known, and, unlike all other great 'charmers', he seemed, and I believe was, entirely unconscious of it. It was, no doubt, partly physical, partly due to the unusual combination of sweetness of nature and affection with rugged intelligence and a complete lack of

> sentimentality, and partly to those personal flavours of the soul which are as unanalysable and indescribable as the scents of flowers or the overtones in a line of great poetry.[12]

In an age of nicknames, he was called 'The Goth', somewhat inappropriately, though after his death in 1906, the nickname itself took on his charisma.

He acted as a catalyst rather than an innovator among his friends, contributing to their mercurial change and interchange of discussion and intellectual development while remaining solidly himself.

Thoby was not without one Stephen weakness; he paid for his sturdiness of character by some unconscious repression: among his letters to his mother from Evelyn's are five from his headmaster, Mr Worsley, describing violent 'attacks', sometimes during bouts of influenza. He had to be moved because his screams frightened the younger boys. There is talk of bars put across the dormitory windows. On one occasion, before the nurse could get to him, he had crashed halfway through an unprotected window. These alarming episodes seem to have subsided: there is no mention of them at Clifton, though when he fell ill he was seriously affected; he nearly died from pneumonia after being sent home too soon after a bout of influenza.

Though he read widely, Thoby was not dedicated to his studies to the extent that Saxon Sydney-Turner and Leonard Woolf were. He loved open-air activities, beagling, riding, hunting; in the Stephen tradition he was a formidable cross-country walker. He had always been a serious naturalist. At school he had kept caterpillars, observing their metamorphoses. Not for him, on visits to the Bristol zoo, the banalities of camels and great cats; he made for the insect house, or watched lizards being fed live cockroaches, carefully counting the ones that got away. Had he read Natural Sciences in Part II of his tripos he might have found an occupation more congenial than the law.

Thoby had a profound influence on Adrian, healthy while he lived, psychologically destructive after his death. I imagine the two brothers, at the beginning of Adrian's first term at Trinity, descending the steps into Great Court each in his own way distinguished with a masculine beauty, Thoby's strong, clean-cut profile favouring the Stephen side of the family, Adrian's more sensitive features and expression recalling his mother's side;

[12] *Sowing: An Autobiography of the Years 1880–1904*

Thoby, six feet two, robust and broad-shouldered, Adrian three inches taller, already a little bowed.

They met at play-reading and debating societies in which Thoby took an active part. These gatherings covered a range of serious play-reading and debate leavened with high-spirited undergraduate humour. At the 300th meeting of the Trinity College Shakespeare Society Thoby read Ferdinand in a reading of *The Tempest* preceded by a dinner on May 29, 1902. Now, reread in heavy volumes in the penumbra of Trinity's Wren Library, the records lose flavour. But there can be no doubt those evenings in one another's smoked-filled rooms were important; and when prolonged till dawn by a few chosen friends, became of overriding significance as they discussed truth, beauty, love, sexual freedom, friendship, and the philosophy of G. E. Moore.

In April 1903, Virginia wrote to Violet Dickinson from Chilworth, Surrey: 'Adrian and Thoby are here. Adrian goes tomorrow but Thoby stays till Sunday. He is a charming great articulate creature with torrents of things shut up in him. Adrian bubbles away, 15 years younger than the rest of us. He grows too fast to think or feel, or do anything else than eat.'

In November 1903 she writes: 'Adrian and his rooms are a cheerful sight. I feel a great affection for him, poor little boy.' (That 'poor little boy' is a recurrent refrain. Adrian was twenty years old; but the early family view persisted. Did Adrian fall in with it, perhaps encourage it to gain affection, attention, or a show of convenient dependence?)

In a letter dated December 1903, Virginia writes that her father has to undergo an operation for cancer; but there was no doubt his disease was terminal. 'Adrian is here – poor little boy – he had guessed nothing but is terribly upset, though he hardly says anything.' Adrian had been with the family at Hindhead when his father's condition was first diagnosed in April 1902. In 1903 he had been at Fritham when they had had to return early. How could he have been ignorant? The death of an unloved parent is more damaging than grief for a loved parent's death; it is possible that he had blocked off his conscious mind to the unbearable truth: that his unconscious wish for his father's death was now to be fulfilled in reality.

Leslie Stephen underwent an operation on December 11, and returned home on January 6, 1904. He lingered on, bearing his condition stoically and courageously, Virginia his chief assistant and companion, till his death on February 22, 1904. The funeral was at the crematorium, Golders Green.[13]

As soon as the Stephen family could escape from the tributes and effusive condolences from family and friends that followed Sir Leslie's death, George Duckworth, who more than ever wanted to prove himself the head of the house and their protector, took them all to Manorbier, on a wild and desolate stretch of the Pembroke coast. Even there they were pursued by a flood of letters and obituary notices that follow the death of a distinguished man of letters, the brunt of which was borne by Virginia. But the place suited them, the air was stimulating and they relived the freedom of body and spirit they had known at St Ives. They began to plan their removal from Hyde Park Gate, a venture initiated by Vanessa who lost no time in investigating Bloomsbury, ignoring the disapprobation of her friend Kitty Maxse and the more peremptory opposition of their conventional Fisher cousins.

They longed to travel, and while still at Manorbier a plan was made to go to Venice. The enthusiasm was intense, Thoby and Adrian could hardly contain themselves. 'Adrian is wildly excited – talks of nothing but Venice and gondolas. This is the right spirit. You can't think how amicable we all are together. . . . We go our own ways and meet fresh and cheerful.'

April 1904 found them at the Grand Hotel in Venice. Gerald Duckworth was with them, not the brightest of companions. But 'Thoby and Adrian are rampant with excitement. Adrian wants to settle here for ever.' They travelled homewards via Florence. 'Adrian and I sang paeans of praise at the top of the San Miniato.'

Adrian returned to Cambridge on April 20. Thoby departed on a walking tour and the others went on to Siena and Genoa, thence to Paris where Thoby rejoined them.

In May Virginia suffered her second serious breakdown, at first under the care of the family doctor, the rigorous Savage. Later she was able to stay with Violet Dickinson for three months where she contracted scarlet fever. She was well enough to rejoin the family in late August at Teversal House, Nottinghamshire, but not to attend George Duckworth's marriage in September to Lady Margaret Herbert at Dulverton in Somerset. The train journey from

[13] The introduction of cremation was fiercely opposed, and Sir Leslie in choosing to be cremated was in the van of enlightened opinion. After a long history of debate and controversy, in and out of Parliament, regulations were finally laid down by the Home Secretary in 1903. But its legality had been established in 1884 in a curious case heard at the Cardiff Assizes by Mr Justice Stephen (Leslie's brother Fitzjames Stephen) who directed the jury that to burn a dead body instead of burying it was not an offence unless it was done so as to amount to a public nuisance.

Nottingham to Somerset was complicated: at one junction Adrian, now typecast as an amiable bungler, mislaid his and Vanessa's luggage.

In October at the beginning of the Michaelmas term, 1904, Virginia, staying with her aunt in Cambridge, writes that Adrian came in 'like a vigorous Daddy-long-legs and brings a breath of fresh air into the place'.

In 1904 the Stephens spent a carefree enjoyable Christmas at Lyndhurst in the New Forest, walking and following buckhounds on foot; Thoby and Adrian longed to ride but could not afford the hire of horses. Then Gerald (the Duckworths behave like benevolent uncles, not always appreciated) sent them £2 10*s.* apiece. So after all the two brothers, suitably mounted, could follow the hunt.

There they are sitting round the fire, the girls footsore after a twelve-mile walk through dead leaves and bogs, the boys stiff from long hours in the saddle. Each has chosen his or her favourite sweet-meat, pink and amber barley sugar and American butter toffee, and sit sucking their long sticks like children in the firelight, perhaps the first and last time they have been or will be together again so intimately and contentedly.

In March 1905, Adrian and Virginia travelled to Portugal and Spain. On April 5 sailing down the Spanish coast, Virginia wrote to Violet Dickinson: 'Adrian is very happy, and takes great care of me, and does my hair at night, and fastens my dress.' From Oporto they travelled on to Seville and Granada. That sea journey was the source of her inspiration for the early chapters of her first novel, *The Voyage Out.* Adrian then returned for his last term at Trinity.

Adrian's time at Cambridge was not untypical of the life of an average undergraduate, with one singular exception: his fondness for hoaxes. Here his talent for acting, his knack of inspired improvisation and his gift for organisation, together with his hatred of pomposity and officialdom, found happy expression. He writes in his book, *The Dreadnought Hoax*, published in 1936, that he and his friend Horace Cole 'had already played some hoaxes on a small scale'. He and Cole, he suggested, should get hold of German Army officers' uniforms and take them to some town near the Franco-German frontier in Alsace-Lorraine. There, suitably dressed, they were to 'take command of some troops and march with them across the frontier into France . . . I had no doubt, of course, that the French would stop us before we had gone a kilometre. We should have surrendered immediately, and perhaps been interned, there would, I hoped, have been . . . an "international incident", the Kaiser would have made gestures and sent telegrams, and other people might have been amused.' Quentin Bell suggests that this was characteristic of Adrian's recklessness: 'Suppose the French had opened fire.'

Cole's plan, being easier and cheaper, was chosen. The Sultan of Zanzibar was visiting England at the time, and it seemed easy enough to impersonate him and pay a state visit to Cambridge. However, a photograph of the Sultan had appeared in the newspapers, so they thought it best to impersonate the Sultan's imaginary uncle and his suite. As they did not want to be sent down, they chose to hoax the mayor rather than the university authorities. Horace Cole played the uncle, two of their friends and Adrian were his suite and, since they meant to have an interpreter less likely to be recognised, an Oxford friend was roped in. They went to London, were made up at a theatrical costumier's, and sent off a telegram to the mayor warning him to expect them. Looking at the photograph of the hoaxers in Adrian's book it seems impossible that they should not have been rumbled – Adrian's enormous height and distinctive appearance alone must surely have given them away. But 'everything went off perfectly'. They were met at the station by the Town Clerk and driven to the Guildhall where they were received by the mayor. 'We then paid a royal visit to a charity bazaar where "the Sultan's uncle" made enormous purchases . . . and were shown round the principal colleges.'

They were conducted back to the station, 'and then arose the problem of escape, for we had no wish to return to London. We entered what was then the Great Eastern part of the station, lifted our skirts, fled through the crowds waiting for the train, out of the Great Northern entrance, jumped into hansoms and . . . told them to drive for all they were worth into the country', whence they made their way across the fields, changed their clothes at a friend's house and returned to their colleges.

They would never have been discovered but for Cole's appetite for publicity. A full account of the escapade was published in the *Daily Mail*. Adrian later heard that the mayor of Cambridge had asked for the culprits to be sent down. The Vice-Chancellor advised the mayor for the sake of his own reputation to think it over. 'In the end nothing happened to us . . . and the hoax was generally felt to be amusing even by people who hotly disapproved of the later hoax on the navy. The person hoaxed was only a Cambridge tradesman (he kept a chemist's shop), whereas naval officers, as one critic said, were "different" – they were "men of honour".'

On June 18, 1905, Virginia writes from 46 Gordon Square that they had been to Adrian's May Week Ball at Trinity. They had picnicked up the river, lunched with Clive Bell, dined with Adrian and danced, no doubt, until dawn – though Vanessa smoked cigarettes instead of dancing. 'Poor Adrian was beginning to feel that his Cambridge was over, and we had to say goodbye to his rooms. It is rather sad that he must give up being taught – or rather, amused – for ever, and earn his own living. He took a third – so at any rate he has his degree, though not a brilliant one.'

Adrian read History for Part I, in 1904, but was excused from taking the examination, possibly because he had begun reading Law. In 1904 he took a Law Special, Part I, and got a Second. In 1905 he took a Law Special, Part II, and got a Third. He had read for an ordinary, not honours degree.

Either before or just after leaving Cambridge, Adrian contracted tertiary syphilis from a woman prostitute. This was common enough at the time and would not be recorded here except that it gives coherence to otherwise random complaints about his behaviour, and his various indispositions. For the first three months the disease is highly infective; but after that, though the symptoms disappear, spirochaetes (bacteria) live on in other organs of the body. It is usually many years before they emerge to cause further symptoms, specially involving the heart.[14]

[14] Information from Sir Benedict Hoskyns, Bt.

7

ST IVES AND GREECE

1905–1906

In October 1904 the Stephens had moved into 46 Gordon Square, the antithesis of Hyde Park Gate, with tall windows that let in the light, completely redecorated by Vanessa with white walls, and with fabrics, curtains and carpets chosen by her. Everyone had their own rooms. Their needs were provided by Sophia Farrell and her staff. She had been cook in Julia's day and now occupied the happy position of an experienced domestic servant indispensable to a family she had seen grow up and had made her own.

George Duckworth was married and Gerald was in rooms elsewhere. By midsummer 1905 Thoby and Adrian were both at home working for exams. Thoby wrote to Leonard Woolf, 'I am now a hard-working law student. I shall publish a book soon on London ornithology.' Virginia had sufficiently recovered to continue her Greek lessons and to give a weekly class on history and English literature at Morley College. She had had her first articles and reviews published, one for the *Guardian*[15] and was an increasingly regular reviewer for the *Times Literary Supplement.* In April 1906 Vanessa had her first commission and went to Sussex to paint Lord Robert Cecil's portrait.

Thoby began holding his 'Thursday Evenings' in 1905, at first chiefly for his Cambridge friends: Lytton Strachey, Walter Lamb, Saxon Sydney-Turner, Clive Bell, and Maynard Keynes. Virginia has related how nonplussed she and Vanessa were at first by their behaviour, so unlike that of the conventional (and boring) young men introduced by George. There they sat smoking their pipes as they had in each other's rooms at Cambridge, oblivious of the presence of the girls, sometimes silent, then, if some cogent observation

[15] The *Guardian*, chiefly circulated among the clergy.

alerted them, breaking into talk. And what talk! Soon Virginia and Vanessa began to see what these uncouths were about: new perspectives opened up, a new way of living and thinking; no subject was barred and, before long, no sexual expression less than explicit. Soon the Stephen girls ventured into discussion, gratified when their observations were considered by one young man or another.

Adrian, like his father before him, was not much interested in philosophical or speculative discussion for its own sake. Nor was he concerned with the nature of love, truth and friendship, or new codes of moral behaviour based on or justified by the theories and principles set forth by G. E. Moore in *Principia Ethica.* Adrian was not wholly enamoured of Moore or his philosophy. As he later commented to his nephew, Quentin Bell, Moore was a less impressive figure than he was thought to be by Thoby's Cambridge friends. Lytton Strachey and other Apostles were shocked by Adrian's rejection of Moore, Adrian told his uncle.

A slightly older Trinity friend joined the group, Desmond MacCarthy, whose brilliant talk was tempered by a geniality that made him beloved by everyone. He was expected to become a writer of importance – a novelist, perhaps. In fact he always was a writer, a distinguished journalist and critic who left five volumes of literary and dramatic criticism, but never the great work hoped for.

By the time Adrian came down for good, 'Thursday Evenings' were a regular feature. Older friends were invited such as Kitty Maxse who had been Stella's friend, with her husband, and their Fisher cousins, still deploring the move to Bloomsbury and not reassured by the Cambridge contingent.

The most enigmatic of Thoby's friends was Saxon Sydney-Turner, now in the Treasury. (Leonard Woolf had entered the Colonial Office.) He would sit silent for a whole evening, or, struck by some point raised, enter the talk and deliver a wise, subtle and often tediously lengthy discourse. A story is told about him which is difficult to believe. It seems that George Duckworth brought in his bride on his arm with pride and introduced her to Saxon who was lighting his pipe. He half got up with a token acknowledgement of recognition, his match still alight. This was in marked contrast to the Stephens and Stracheys who though they might cut you, ignore you or allow a fleeting expression of tedium, did so with perfect politeness. Yet Saxon and Adrian formed a close friendship based on their love of music; it was to Saxon that Adrian later wrote long letters while living with Duncan Grant in Lincolnshire, and he was among the guests when, in the summer of 1905, the Stephens took a house in Carbis Bay, Cornwall, the first time they had returned to St Ives since their mother's death. Among the other guests were Gerald Duckworth, Kitty Maxse and her husband, and Jack Hills.

But St Ives was for the family. The night of their arrival they stole up to Talland House in the dark, opened the gate and climbed the familiar steps into the garden. They were invited to tea with the current owners.

In the summer of 1906 the Stephens planned their momentous expedition to Greece and Turkey. Preparations were exhaustive: 'Thoby and Adrian made their wills; boxes and stores, green veils, blue spectacles, white boots, grey felt hats, green-lined umbrellas, paintboxes and easels, medicines and the help of Messrs Thomas Cook had all to be obtained' (Quentin Bell, *Biography of Virginia Woolf*).

The brothers left a month ahead, on August 10, planning to travel via the Balkans and meet Vanessa, Virginia and her friend Violet Dickinson at Olympia. Their journey was adventurous: few Victorian travellers had explored Montenegro, Dalmatia and Albania. On September 17 when they were all assembled in Athens Thoby wrote to Clive Bell (the Stephen brothers were sparing with commas):

> Grand Hotel d'Angleterre
> Athens (Greece)
>
> My Dear Bell
> Your letter to me is in a coat pocket which is in a bag which is derelict somewhere in the Peloponnese; consequently I must write without reference to it in order to catch the mail and must also address this to Melksham. I can't remember if there is anything much to answer – I think not – oh you will be glad to hear that the white umbrellas were broken over Montenegrin horses and the green spectacles have been discarded as useless so the Acropolis is to that extent inviolate. Our itinerary has been roughly this. We went first to Trieste – thence by steamer down the coast of Istria and Dalmatia for 3 or 4 days – a most delightful trip – exquisite sea, perfect weather – charming coast (to employ epithets which come readily to the perusers of guide books) and little towns (we visited two or three a day to load or unload some trifles) where a Venetian palace, or cathedral a Roman temple or amphitheatre a picturesque market or an ancient fort served to distract an hour – the

Venetian architecture of these parts is by the way rather remarkable, some really fine things, and none of them had their air of being sights. At Cattano the southern most town of Dalmatia we landed and drove up to Cetinje the capital of Montenegro. Thence we drove to Niksic the principal other town of the country and there the road comes to an end and we got horses and rode towards the NW frontier and got to the Durmitor mountains, the biggest range in those parts.

The weather was damnable for the first 3 days, food very scant lodgings either the cowshed or family bedroom of some kindly inhabitant but it was extremely jolly notwithstanding – from there we rode back to the coast by another route. The Montenegrins are not without interest. Their appearance in the first place is (the men's) often magnificent (the women's) generally graceful frequently fine. They are as you know the only people in the Balkans who have never caved in to the Turks tho' always at war with them and they have all the virtues of unconquerable mountaineers of romance. Their land is little but stones relieved with a forest and prairie or two in the north but fine in shape and colour. They wear a capital costume which shows off their fine figure and bearing (of which they are fully conscious) very well. In Cetinje they swagger about like the chorus of an opera and leave the work to the women (who by the way always kiss the men's hands and generally know their place). In the country they are odd uncouth-looking barbarians, often of prodigious stature.

I dread the more civilised rougher type – who always go armed with pistol or rifle – though the necessity in the interior at least is not very obvious. They have also tribal bards who chant to an odd primeval instrument which buzzes like a monotonous bee. They are a most interesting crew in many ways and I will describe 'em at length to you you may be sure my boy. From there we went to Corfu and thence to Athens for 4 days – from there we went to Tripolitza in Arcadia and drove through Arcadia to Sparta – rode across Taygetus to the top of the Messenian bay thence up the plains of Messene between Ithene and Taygetus to Elis and Olympia – passing on our way the wonderful temple of Apollo at Bassae – a lovely Doric temple perched on a lonely 4000 foot mountain away from everything – astoundingly fine. Otherwise we visited no antiquities on the way but saw a great deal of country of all kinds of which one can only say that surely such a country deserved to be the home of the Greeks – it is quite unspeakably fine. I have seen nothing comparable to it. At Olympia we met our family and after a couple of days there went on to Corinth and here where we shall be for 5 or 6 days.

My good fellow it is undoubtedly worth it, indeed you must jolly well come as soon as you can and if possible at this time of year when there are next to no trippers and the country is at its best. People talk infernal rot about the heat. We rode most days 12 or 13 hours with ½ hour halt at midday and hardly felt it. The mornings are perfect. We didn't care much for the modern Greek in the Peloponnese – perhaps because we chiefly saw innkeepers and horse dealers but there were some good fellows enough. As for Athens you may possible [*sic*] conceive the Parthenon to be like a dismantled and disreputable British Museum – if so you are singularly in error. For the first place you have no notion of its colour which is many and unutterably divine and secondly you cannot appreciate its shape which is the consummation of human architecture – or divine for that matter. The nobility the grace, the subtlety cannot be dimly adumbrated by any photograph picture or other visibility – but the colour of Athens and Attica by God sir you must come and see it and then your Nunc dimittis if you like – Olympia also is eminently sublime and egad the Hermes – its Virgilian. But just come.

yrs J.T.S. [Julian Thoby Stephen]

Part of their tour round the Peloponnesus may have been by carriage. But for the most part they hired horses. Characteristically, Thoby's laconic itinerary makes light of hardships undergone or the danger of their crossing the 4,000-feet-high Taygetus Mountain Pass. Greece, even in October, is very hot, plains and olive groves parched. Making for the Taygetus Pass they rode from Sparta to Mistra over malaria-breeding marshy ground, viewing the mountain range ahead. The road snakes steeply up the long ascent, folding itself into a vast gorge, on the one hand a bare mountain escarpment, on the other a sheer drop into fathomless green depths of vegetation and forest. On a narrow dirt track the exploit must have been a test of nerve and horsemanship.

The Greek landscape is everywhere on a superhuman scale, great heights, long distances continually marked by the presence of an ancient civilisation, overarched by a cloudless blue sky. To travel through it as Thoby and Adrian did, at one with parched earth, arid rock and reviving shade, unites such travellers in a bond closer than kinship.

When on September 13 they reached Olympia and met the family they found Vanessa unwell. The three women had travelled by train to Brindisi, thence by boat to Patras and by train to Olympia. After two days they all set off for Athens, but the train journey increased Vanessa's indisposition and they had to pause at Corinth for her to rest. In Athens she was sufficiently recovered for them to make a short excursion to Mount Pentelicon, north-east of Athens, famous for its marble quarries. On a longer expedition they sailed to Nauplia, thence to Tyrins, Mycenae and Epidaurus. But the return train journey again upset her; once more they had to stop for a night or two at Corinth before going on to Athens. There she seemed sufficiently recovered to be left with Violet Dickinson while the others visited the Noels at Achmetaga on the Aegean island of Euboea.

The party returned to Athens to find Vanessa 'alarmingly ill'. Virginia, with Violet Dickinson, spent the rest of her time in Athens with the invalid, heating goat's milk over a spirit lamp. The brothers, with scant concern for the invalid or her nurse, after a few days' frustration in the hotel lounge returned to the Peloponnesus. There is some discrepancy between the two accounts in Thoby's first and second letters, but it seems likely that they paid a second visit to Bassae. The 'good walk', '8 stoney miles from the town', was a steep climb along goat tracks up the mountainside, further evidence of their stamina. From there they returned to Corinth and Delphi.

Thoby's second letter to Clive Bell is also from Athens.

Tourist's Palace Hotel
Athens (Greece)
Oct. 10

My dear Bell
I fancy my last letter to you was from here. Since then our

plans have been considerably changed. Vanessa who had been rather unwell for some time turned out to have appendicitis. She is now convalescent but won't be able to leave for a week at least and it's probable that we shall have to give up Constantinople and we mayn't be back till the beginning of Nov. Possibly tho' I shall try and get back before. On leaving here we went to Aegina where Adrian and I had a good walk to one of the best temples going most magnificently placed (the Greeks by the way obviously selected the sites for their temples with an eye to beauty alone – this for instance is 8 stoney miles from the town). Bassae is on the top of a desolate mountain where there is also a museum with some things dug up this year, not yet arranged or classified but some to my mind first class. Thence by boat to Nauplia from where we did Epidaurus (an astonishing fine theatre there). Tiryns (Cyclopean business really fine) Mycenae (most uncommonly noble) and on to Corinth. From there Adrian and I went to Delphi – perhaps the most wonderful place in Greece except Athens. Apart from the admirable sculptures in the museum there and the exquisite remains of temples etc the place is probably the most beautiful going.

It is as you know placed in a great cleft on a spur of Parnassus 2000 feet up with a noble prospect – not distractingly wide – below of a valley [*sic*] of olive woods sloping to a crescent bay and the Gulf of Corinth and Achaean mountains beyond. From the chasm above the precinct flows the Castalian fount down a ravine. You can imagine my delight when from the great cliffs above there sailed to complete the magnificence of the spectacle 5 whopping griffon vultures, 2 golden eagles, many ravens and above all a lammergeier. This last is one of the noblest birds that fly, larger even than a griffon – a golden eagle is a pigmy to it. It's shaped rather like a falcon than a vulture or eagle with its long pointed wings and wedged tail. Its colour is almost white in the sunshine and with my glasses I could distinctly see the black moustache. It is something of a rarity and pleased me uncommonly.

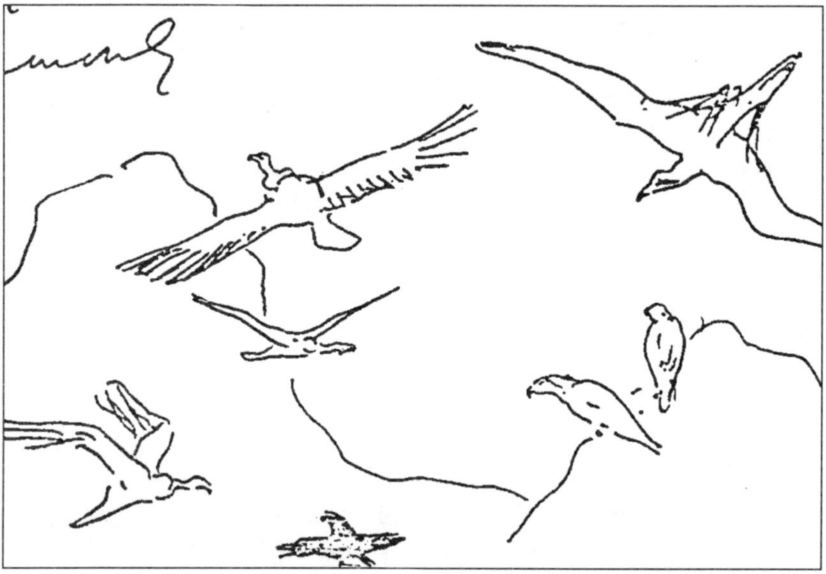

(This hasn't quite come off I'm afraid.)

From there we went on to Euboea to stay with the Noels. The father of the present owner bought an estate there just after the war of Greek Independence. The present owner has been there all his life and hardly ever leaves it. His son and daughter spend a good deal of time in England. It is a most delightful place in fine country and has various unexcavated primaeval remains in the neighbourhood and a magnificent coast a few miles off. Unfortunately we only had 2–3 days there. Well this is the end of my paper. God be with you.

J.T.S.

After a fortnight Thoby returned to England, leaving the others to continue their journey to Constantinople. But Vanessa, who had been unwell throughout their tour, collapsed and had to be carried off the boat at Constantinople. They returned to England by train. At Dover they were met by George Duckworth with a nurse for Vanessa. They found Thoby ill in bed at 46 Gordon Square with a high temperature.

Virginia found herself with two invalids to tend. Her dearest friend, Violet, was also gravely ill at her own home. Living, as she described herself, 'in the midst of nurses, bedpans, carbolic and doctors', Virginia managed with her usual admirable good sense when faced, as so often, with illness. Vanessa's illness was never diagnosed; but it seems possible that she was suffering from typhoid; Thoby's reference to 'appendicitis', suggesting inflammation of the bowel, is significant.

Thoby's illness, pain and exhaustion were perhaps exacerbated by his being mistreated for malaria before he was found to have typhoid. The family were naturally outraged, specially as the ubiquitous Dr Savage was at first in charge. But for the first ten days the symptoms are similar and a differential diagnosis could only have been made by sophisticated tests which were not available at that time. And malaria was known to be endemic in parts of Greece. Before the advent of antibiotics treatment for typhoid was based on rigorous isolation and nursing care. The outcome was often fatal.

'Thoby passed from crisis to crisis; he became listless, weary and weak; all he had left at the end was the courage to die bravely' (Quentin Bell, *Biography of Virginia Woolf*).

The reaction of Thoby's Cambridge friends to his death was at first incredulity. Lytton Strachey saw the announcement in *The Times.* Saxon Sydney-Turner wrote to them all: 'The Goth is dead.' And so the word went round: the unbelievable loss had to be taken in, their mourning shared. A week after his death, Vanessa and Virginia invited Lytton Strachey and Clive Bell to see them. There was no mention of Adrian, who, presumably, was in the house. But Saxon wrote that he had been with Adrian and Virginia most days.

When I asked Ann Synge, Adrian's daughter, about Thoby's death, she replied in a harsh, sad voice that seemed to echo her father's: 'The wrong man died.'

They hadn't said so? No, but they made him feel it.

There is Adrian's own guilt, common in all bereavement, to be weighed up, and how much he might have projected it onto the behaviour of family and friends. Nevertheless, it seems probable that they did indeed feel just that; and Adrian's isolation, partly self-induced, was a burden added to his grief.

Two days after Thoby's death Clive Bell, who had long wished to marry Vanessa, had twice proposed and been refused, was accepted: they became engaged, and were married in February 1907. Thus, Adrian and Virginia were left to continue their life together.

It has become an accepted cliché that Adrian was 'overshadowed' by Thoby. This may have been the view of others; but there is no evidence that Adrian himself felt so. Of the two it is Thoby who might have harboured some latent resentment, remembering their mother's marked preference for her younger son. But this would have been uncharacteristic of his generous openheartedness. After their father's death he had taken his place among the four young Stephens. Equally Adrian had his part in family life, looking up to Thoby and sharing in their fond admiration. So long as Thoby lived their uncomplicated affectionate relationship gave Adrian confidence and an assured role. With Thoby's death he lost the surest most stable figure of his life. Then it may have been that he became 'overshadowed' – by Thoby's memory.

For Virginia and Adrian their brother's death was irreparable. Virginia had her own way of immortalising him in *Jacob's Room* and in *The Waves.* For Adrian there was no such release. But the recent discovery among the papers preserved by his daughters, Ann and Judith, reveals his own characteristic way of perpetuating Thoby's memory: an album of photographs, meticulously captioned. In my mind's eye I see him in some dark, red-blinded room holding up negative after dripping negative. Here is their steamer moored at the quay at Ravingo: 'JTS' (Thoby) under a sunlit arch at Zara; J.T.S in the carriage they hired from Cattaro to Cetinje; Stanko Jojovitch their Montenegrin guide through that 'stoney land', their long legs astride small, stout ponies, the two of them riding between Sparta and Calamata; views of the temple of Bassae; 'Embarking our beasts on the ferry-boat' at Olympia; the reunited party at Olympia; Virginia and Vanessa on donkeys or mules with their brothers ascending Mount Pentelicon. All is there, sepia-faded with the years, recreating that last journey. And there is a map, traced with a mapping pen on a sheet of writing paper headed 29 Fitzroy Square, the house he and Virginia moved into in April 1907. All the places Thoby named are methodically listed in Adrian's clear, small hand.

8

GORDON SQUARE AND FITZROY SQUARE

1907–1908

From the time of her engagement Vanessa moved away from Virginia and Adrian. She was often absent with Clive Bell visiting friends and introducing each other to their respective relations. Vanessa, Virginia observed, was deliriously happy. At first she felt her sister's engagement as a dereliction, tearing asunder their close companionship; nor did she feel Clive Bell to be an adequate husband for Vanessa. It took time, and Vanessa's patient persuasion, for her to accept that marriage did not mean too harrowing a change; they would live near by, see each other often. When they were apart they wrote to each other daily. Adrian felt no such deprivation. Of all Thoby's friends, Clive had been the easiest to get on with. They shared the same enjoyment in country pursuits; and Clive's intelligent sophistication appealed to his future brother-in-law.

In any case Adrian's depression and complicated burden of grief and guilt would have cut him off from responding fully to any external event. He must have been poor company for Virginia, and no support during the month following Thoby's death. Not that he was prostrated or idle; like a true Stephen he worked: his final law examinations were due the following year. Virginia, too, worked, teaching English Literature and History at Morley College, reading, writing articles and beginning to experiment, to write for herself.

Her chief desire was to recreate Thoby, to learn more of that part of his life lived away from home, his time at Cambridge. She was jealous of those who had shared his life and envious on her own account of the experience from which women were barred. She wanted to see no one but his Cambridge friends, Lytton Strachey, Clive, and Saxon Sydney-Turner, who mourned with her but could not, for all their sympathy, help her in this respect. Perhaps one of them could write about him? They tried, but failed. Their problem was insoluble: asked by Thoby's sister to recreate the man they adored, who had been the centre of an essentially masculine group in an exclusively masculine environment they were unable to respond.

In spite of her grieving, Virginia's first care was for Adrian. She wrote to Violet Dickinson: 'You are one of the few people – Adrian is another – who make it worth while to live and be happy.' She frequently writes to Violet and to another friend, Madge Vaughan, of how she wants to make him happy, 'poor little boy' (Adrian was twenty-three). It was at least partly for his benefit that they spent Christmas 1906, in the same house, near Lyndhurst, where they had all been so happy together the previous year.

Violet showered her with presents. And there was a cheque for Adrian. He was doubtful about accepting it but, as Virginia wrote, it would be 'enough for five days' hunting, nothing he cares for more. Will keep him out all day, poor little boy.' Though severe weather prevented hunting, they were contented enough in spite of the sadness of mutual recollections, going for walks, scuffing dead, frost-curled leaves, glimpsing a deer through the bare trees, Adrian treading ice in frozen ruts. At night they sat over the fire reading, or talking over the future. 'It really begins to look quite vigorous and healthy.' Adrian brewed whisky toddy over the fire, 'shouting out stories of father when he was an undergraduate'. She goes on, 'It is a blessing to have that book.[16] I think Fred knew that.'

For the New Year they joined Vanessa and Clive at his family home at Seend in Wiltshire. The house and his family were what Virginia found most alien: 'a rich and illiterate house, set in its own grounds, Gothic, barbaric. I dip my pen into the hoof of an old hunter. . . . The daughters are so exactly what one would have guessed. . . . They play hockey and beagle. . . . The girls come down to dinner in pale blue satin with blue satin bows in their hair.'

Adrian, however, brightened up considerably. With beagling and shooting he was on familiar ground. He enjoyed the company of young women, and was a success with the girls, who laughed at his jokes. Similarly, when they visited Charles Booth[17] at Gracedieu Manor in Leicestershire, he felt himself at home. It will be seen that though he enjoyed the stimulating company of the bright spirits who gathered in and around Gordon Square he had a liking

[16] Frederic William Maitland, author of the *Life and Letters of Leslie Stephen*, had just died.

[17] Charles Booth, a writer on social questions, had employed George Duckworth as unpaid secretary, as had Austen Chamberlain.

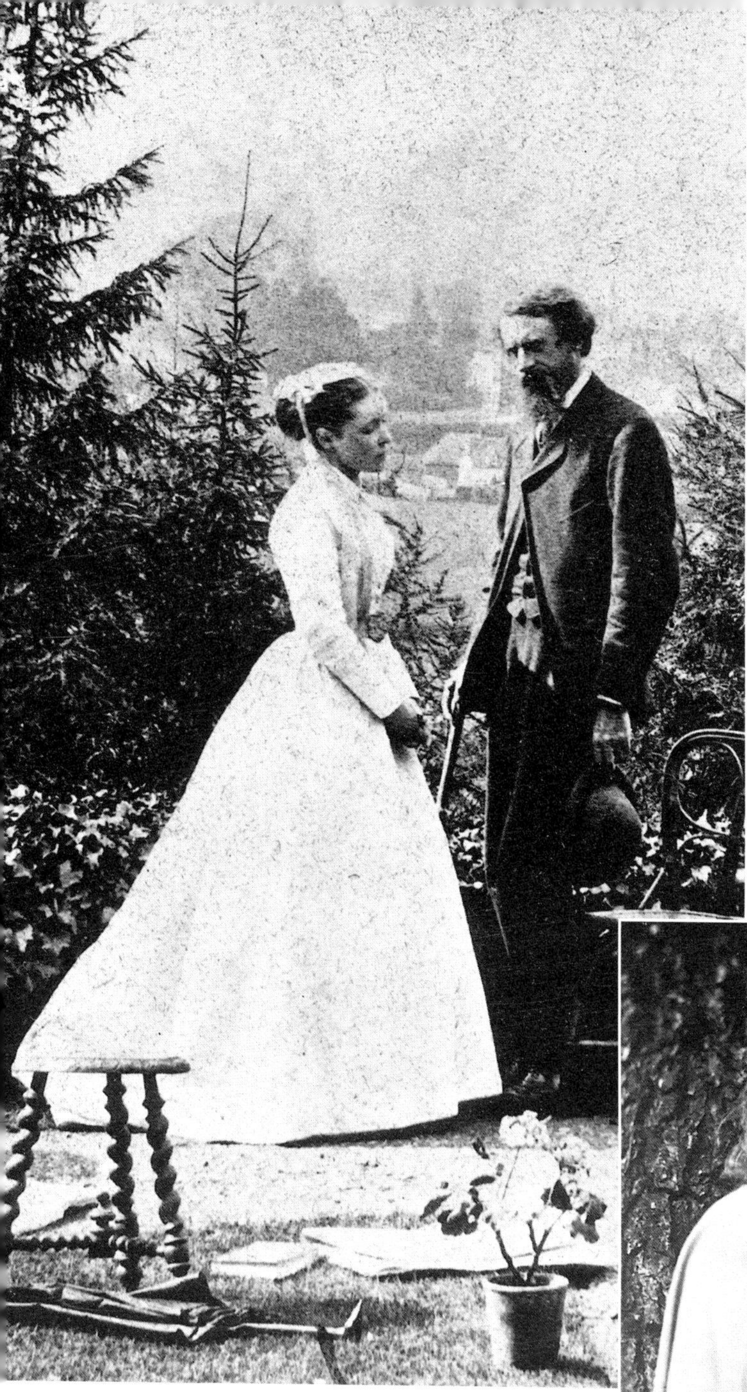

Leslie Stephen and his first wife, Harriet Marian (Minny), Thackeray's daughter. Married 1867. She was peaceful and equable, shared his love of the Swiss Alps. (*Julia Cameron*)

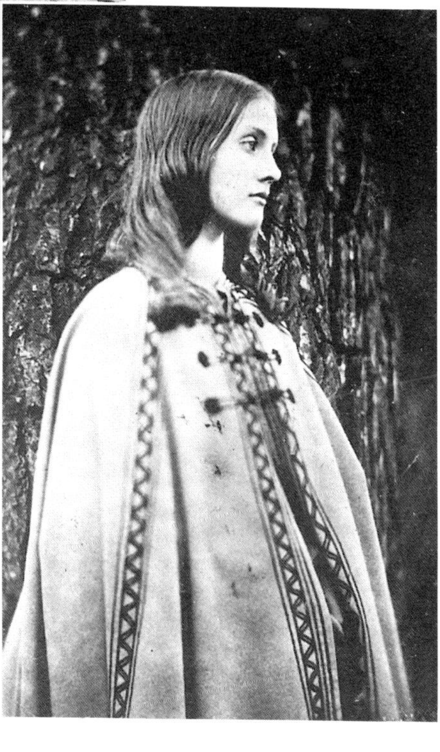

Julia Jackson, Leslie Stephen's second wife. Renowned for her beauty, drawn by G.F. Watts, Edward Burne-Jones used her as a model, her aunt, Julia Cameron, photographed her (as here). From her first marriage she had three children, two sons and a daughter, Stella, who managed the household after Adrian's mother, Julia, died when he was ten.

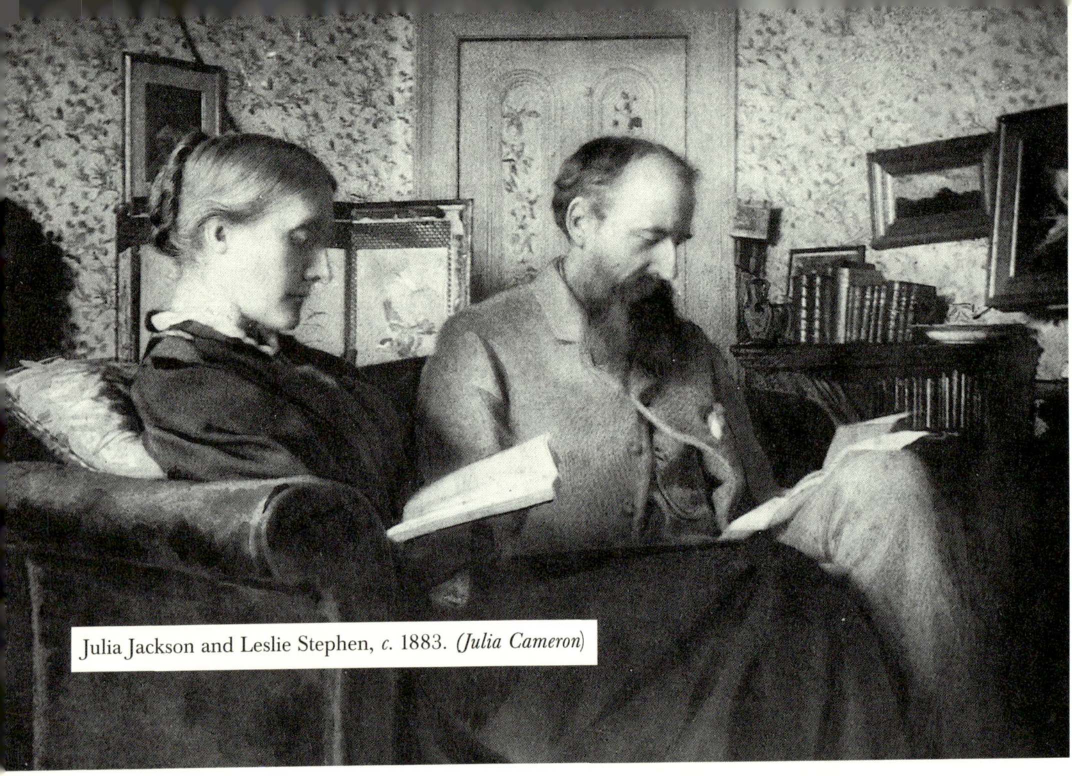

Julia Jackson and Leslie Stephen, *c.* 1883. *(Julia Cameron)*

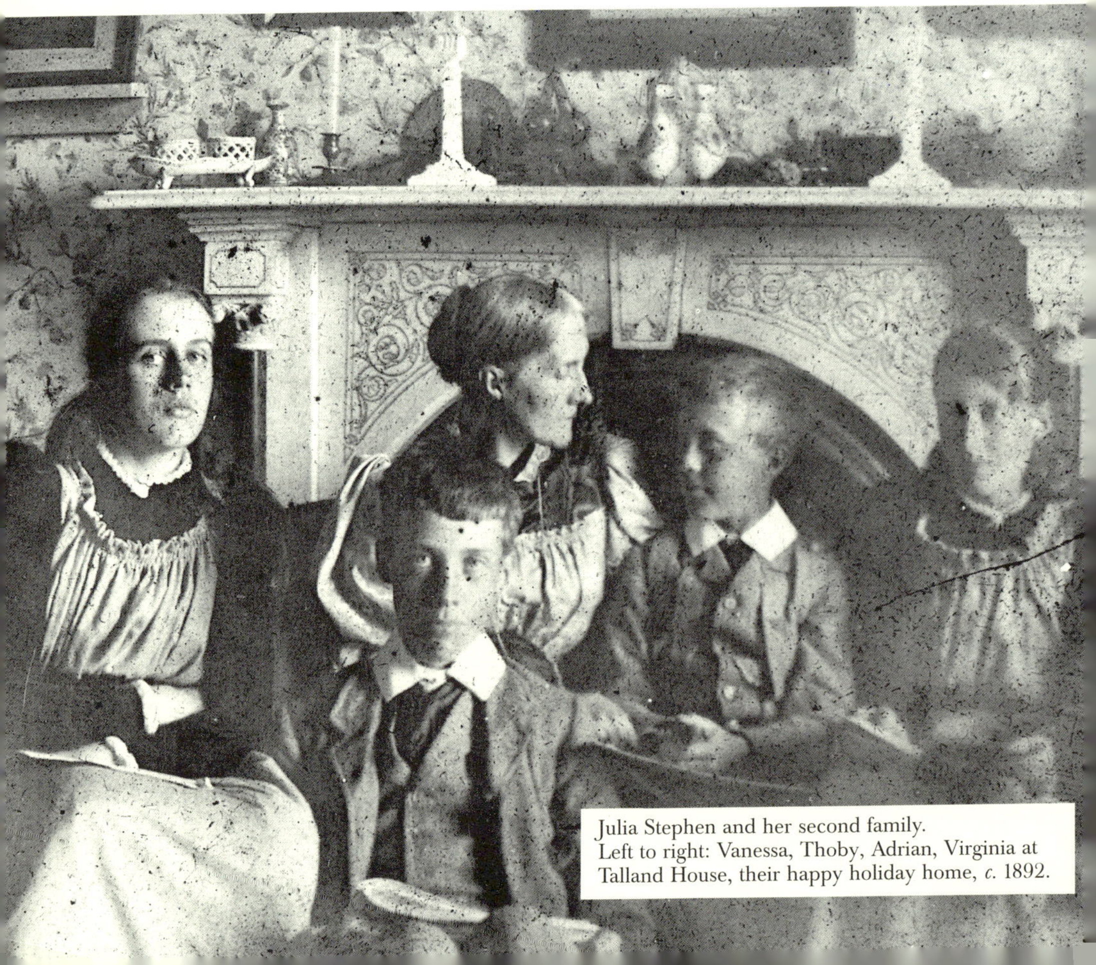

Julia Stephen and her second family.
Left to right: Vanessa, Thoby, Adrian, Virginia at Talland House, their happy holiday home, *c.* 1892.

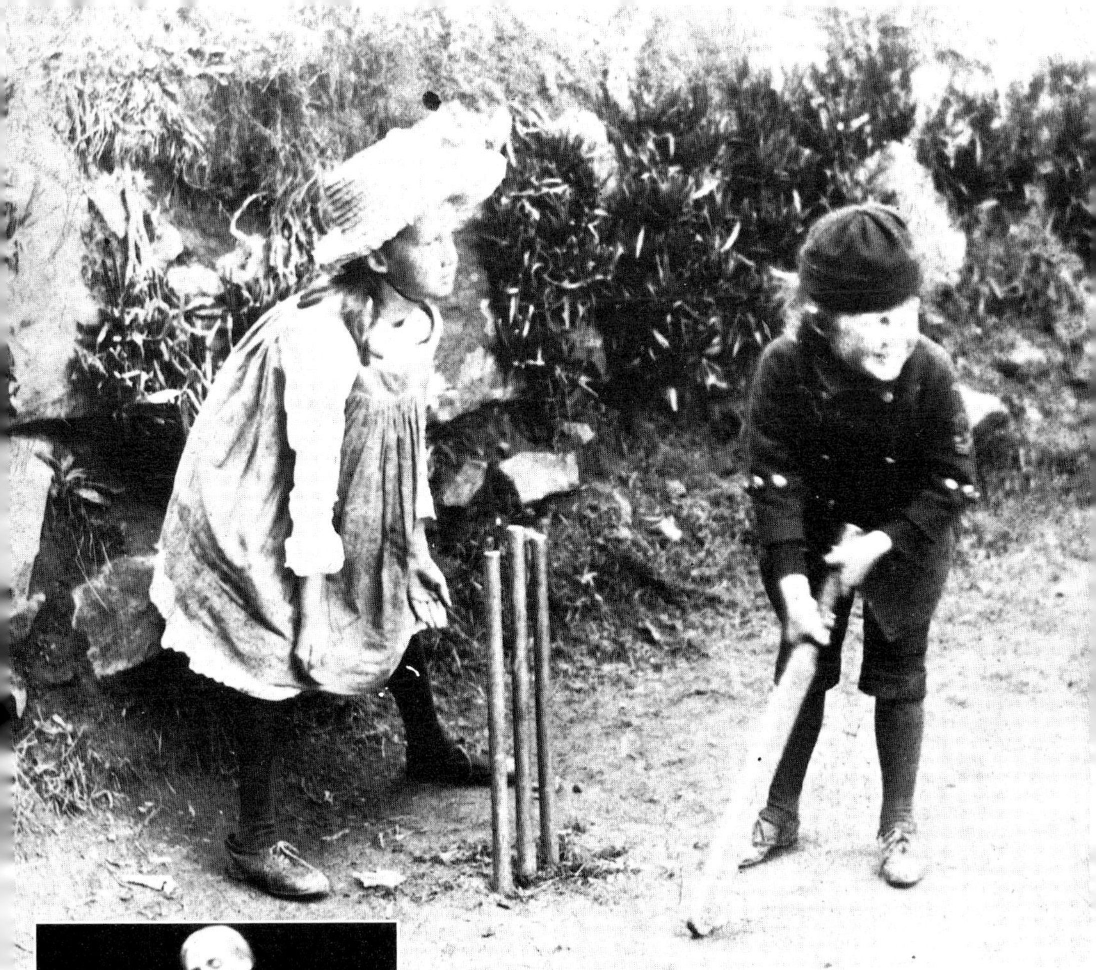

Virginia keeps wicket, with Adrian at the stumps, Talland House, *c.* 1889.

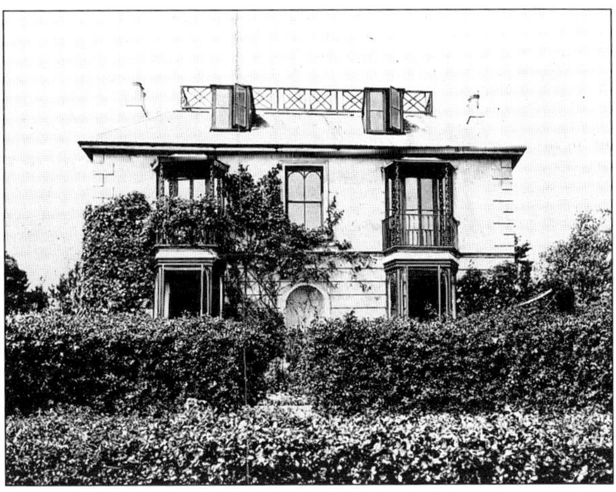

Talland House, St Ives, Cornwall, the setting of Virginia Woolf's *To the Lighthouse* (in which the character, James, was based on Adrian).

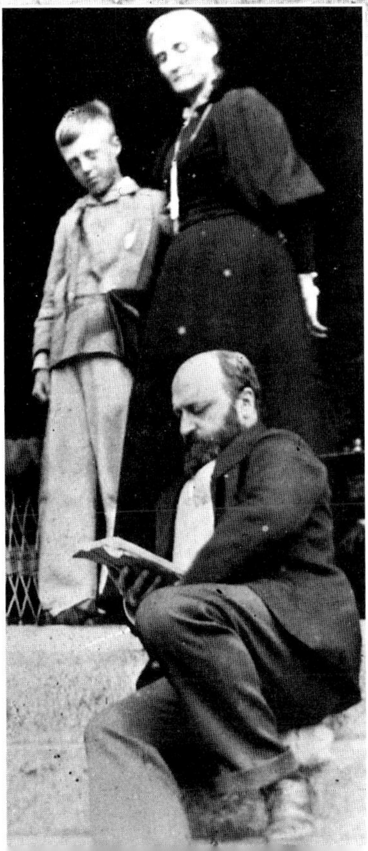

Adrian, Julia, and Henry James.

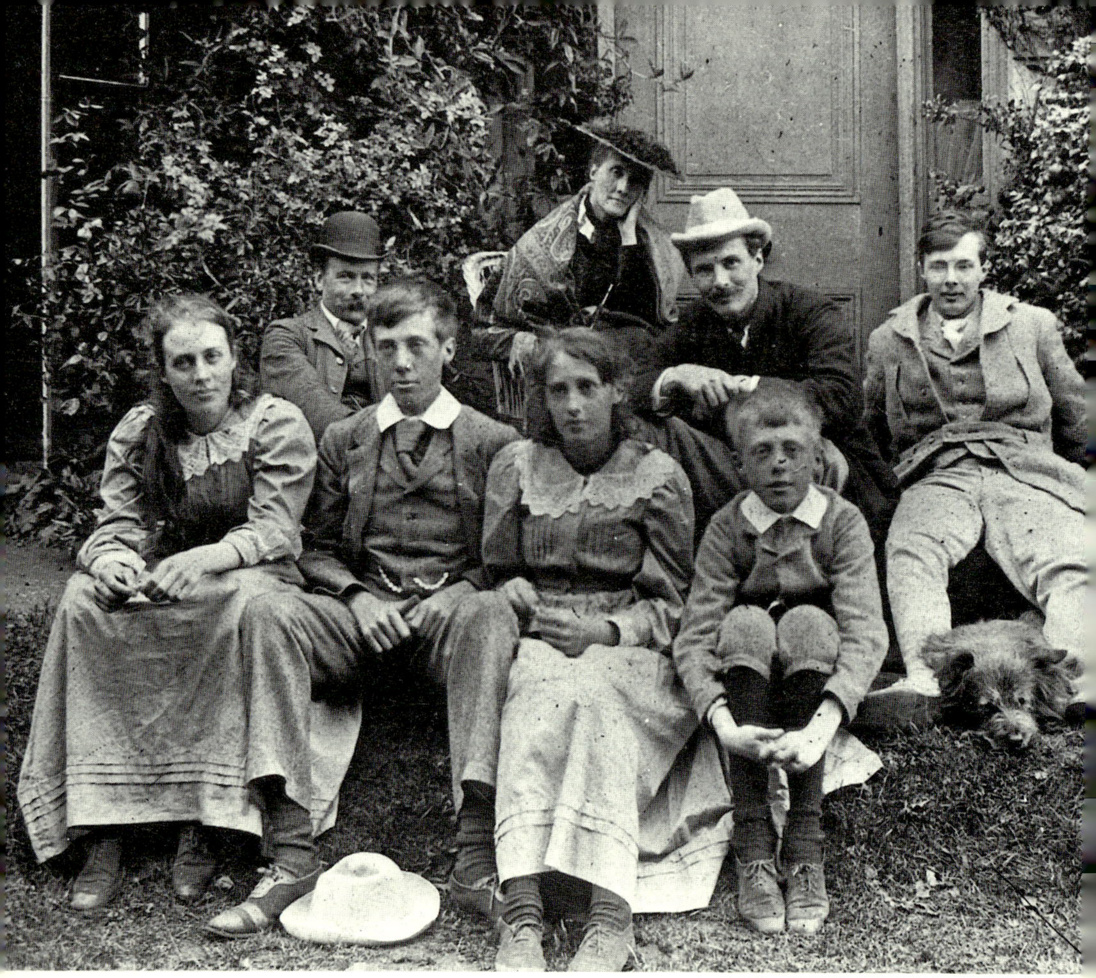

Julia's two families at Talland House. Left and right of Julia: Horatio Bottomley, George Duckworth and Gerald Duckworth. In front, left to right: Vanessa, Thoby, Virginia, Adrian. Stella Duckworth not present. Perhaps she was taking the photograph.

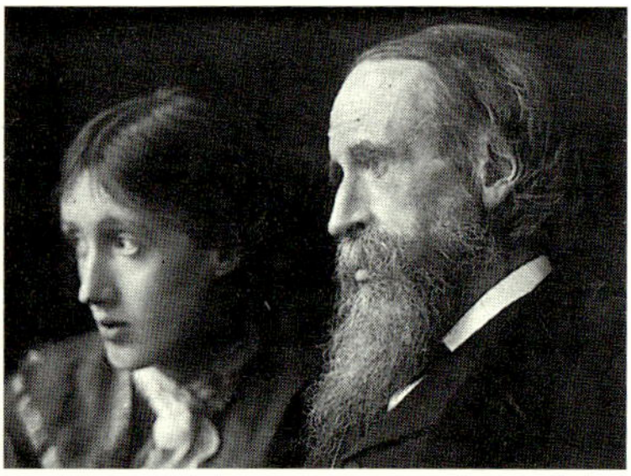

Virginia and Leslie Stephen.

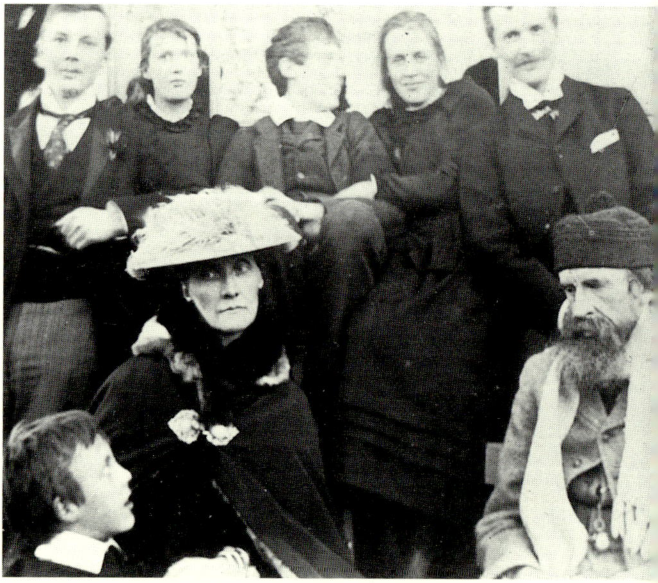

The Duckworths and Stephens, again without Stella (back row, left to right): Gerald, Virginia, Thoby, Vanessa, George. Adrian comforts his mother. Leslie Stephen's exhausted appearance suggests the photograph was taken about 1891, the year he gave up editing the *Dictionary of National Biography* which Julia believed had exhausted him.

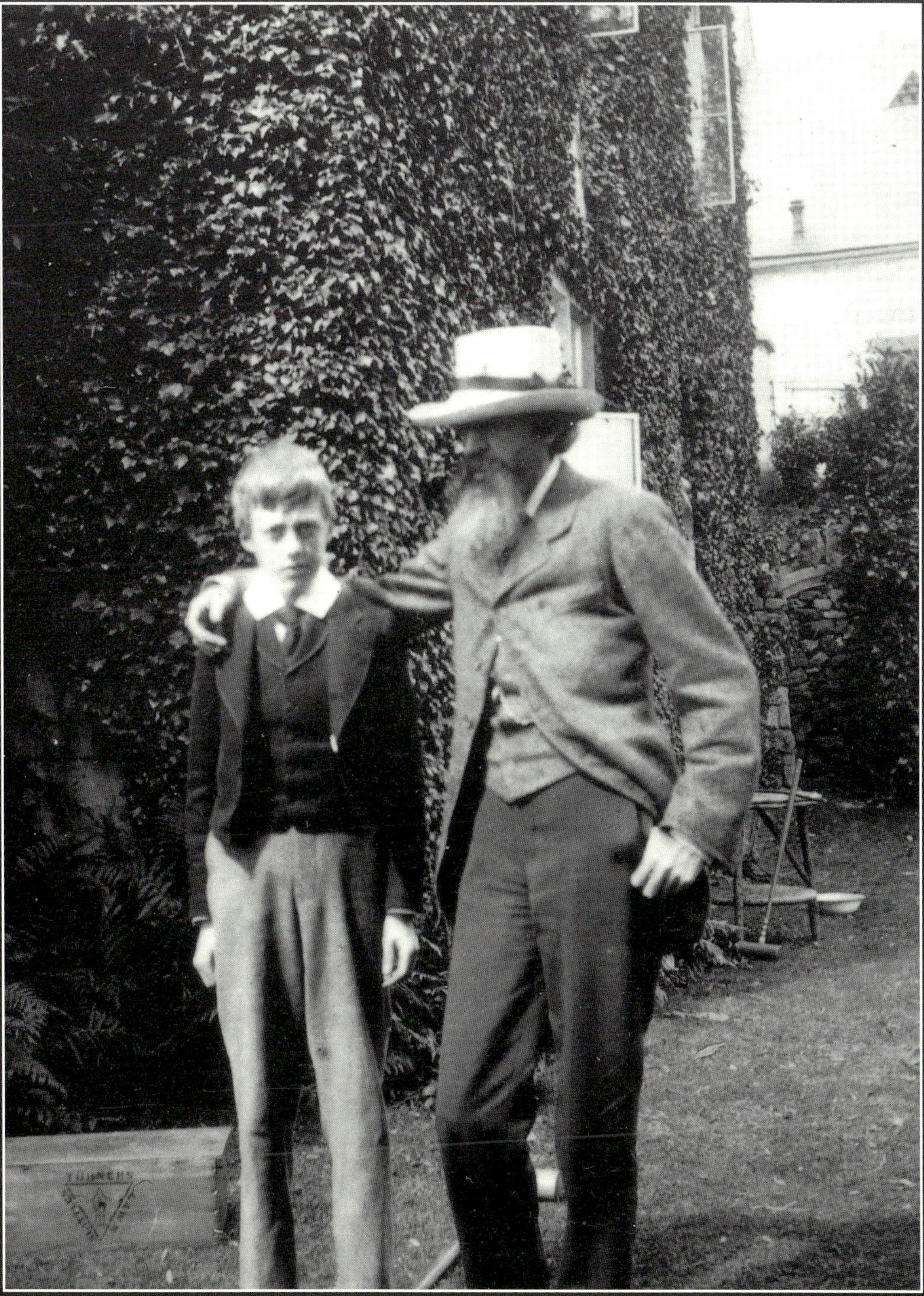

Adrian and Leslie Stephen at the Vicarage, Painswick, Gloucestershire, 1897: 'The elderly father making a tentative gesture . . . the bleak look on Adrian's face.' (see p.22)

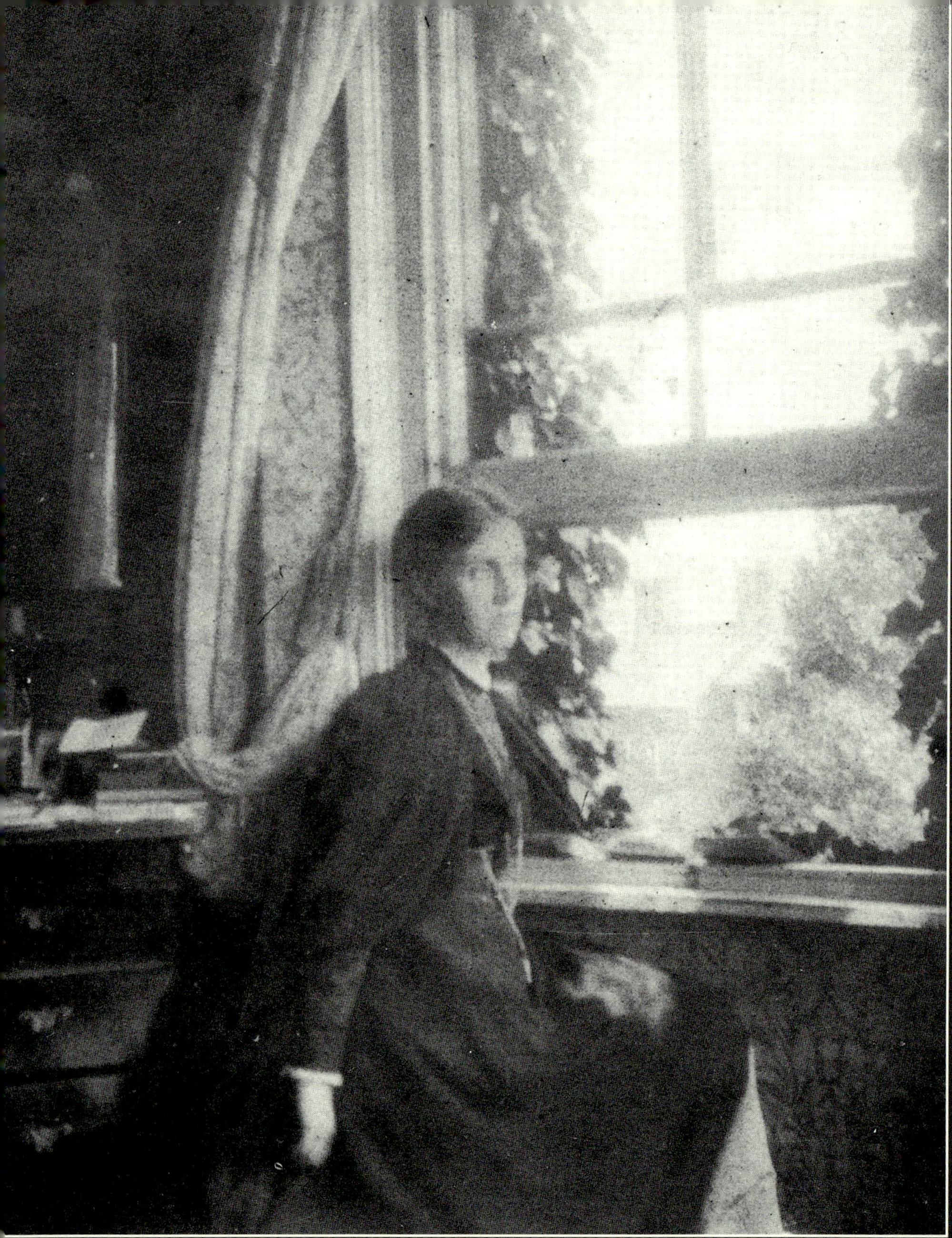

Stella Duckworth at Dimbola, the house at Wimbledon which was owned principally as an investment. She was an important support to Adrian after his mother's death when she took on the formidable duty of keeping the household accounts which had to be presented to Leslie Stephen weekly, making him groan and express fears that he was being bankrupted!

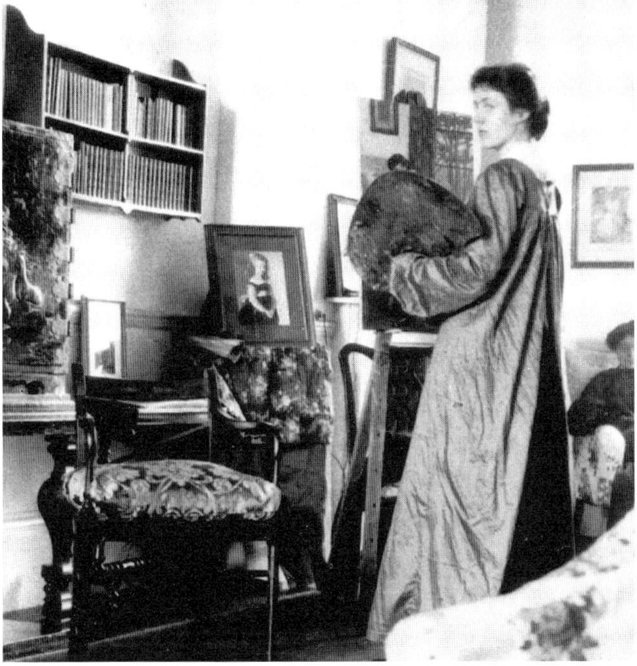

Vanessa painting in the drawing room. She did not have her own studio until she moved the family to Bloomsbury after Sir Leslie's death.

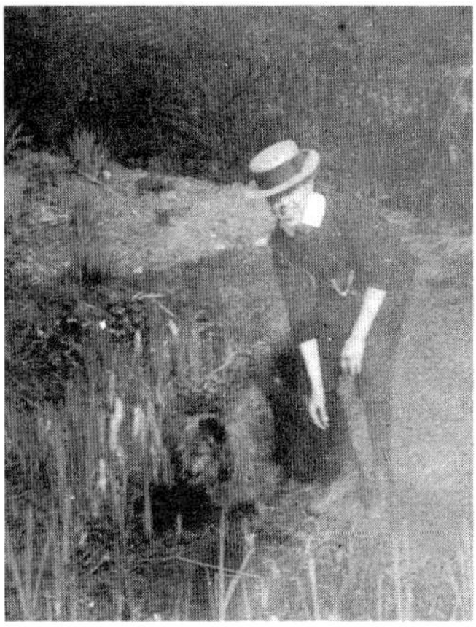

Adrian and the Stephen dog, Shag. He loved dogs and much later in life, in one of his papers, compared an analyst's approach to his patients with that of a man confronted with a savage watch-dog chained to its kennel.

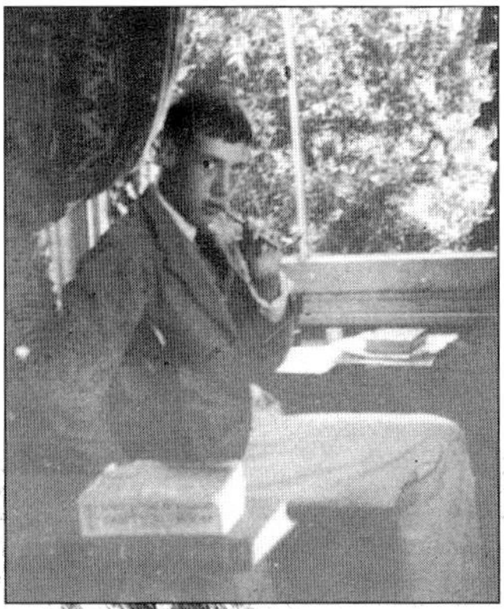

Thoby doing his maths holiday task, on holiday from Clifton.

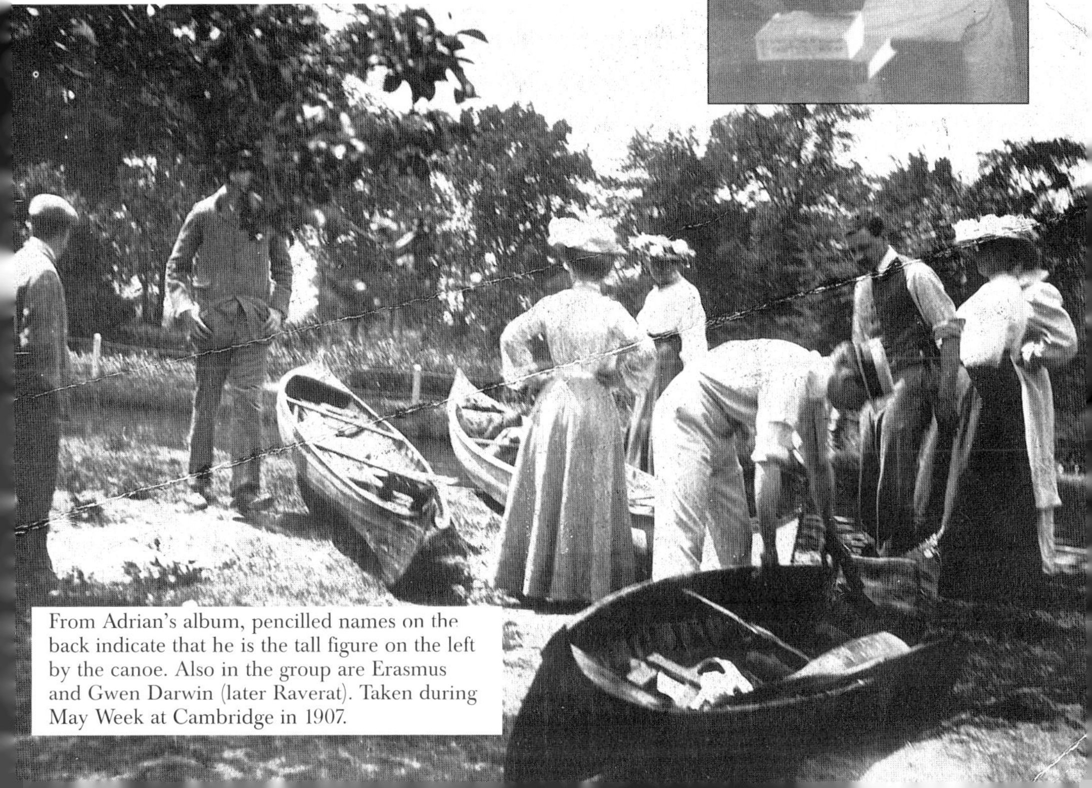

From Adrian's album, pencilled names on the back indicate that he is the tall figure on the left by the canoe. Also in the group are Erasmus and Gwen Darwin (later Raverat). Taken during May Week at Cambridge in 1907.

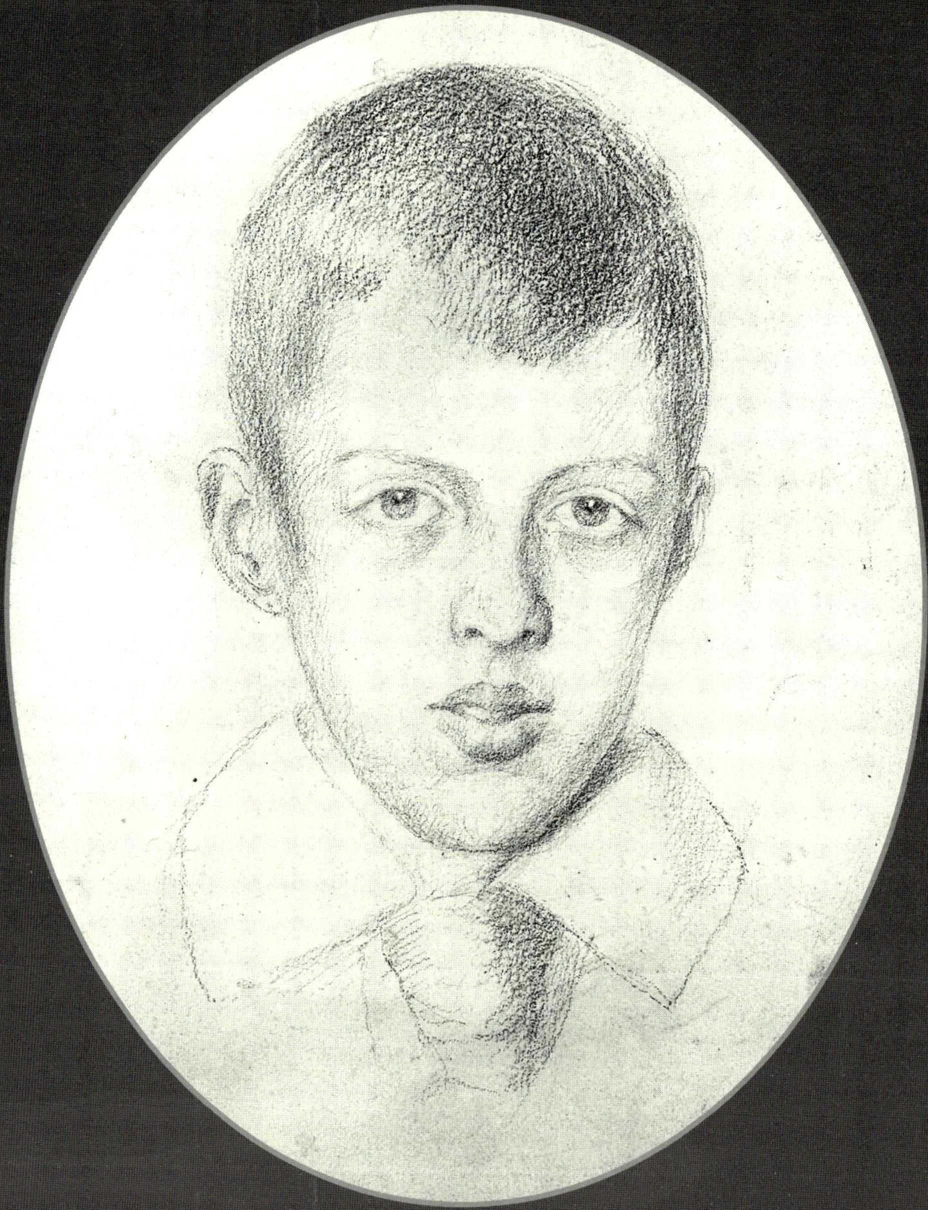

Adrian when at Westminster, by G.F. Watts the celebrated Victorian artist, friend of Julia's parents.

throughout his life for 'ordinary people' such as Horace Cole, whose one distinction was his expertise in 'hoaxes'.

At the beginning of 1907 Virginia was occupied in finding a house for herself and Adrian since Vanessa and Clive were to live in Gordon Square. 'Adrian is perfectly charming . . . I want to make a home for him.' She found 29 Fitzroy Square, W1, where George Bernard Shaw had lived before his marriage. Her conventional friends were even more appalled than they had been when the Stephens had moved into Gordon Square. Fitzroy Square was thought to be a disreputable quarter. And there was the unsuitability of her living with her brother – she needed protection, which Adrian seemed unlikely to provide. But Virginia stuck to her guns, even consulting the police to reassure them.

Adrian and Sophia Farrell, she said, entirely approved. 'Sophie, who was very stout, declared, "I ought to be able to cut myself up among the lot of you," adding more gravely, "but it must be Miss Virginia; she's such a harum-scarum thing she wouldn't know if they sold her. She don't know what she has on her plate."'[18] The house was delightful, near enough to Gordon Square for constant meetings, yet far enough for independence.

On February 26, Virginia wrote to Violet Dickinson asking if Adrian could come down to her in Hertfordshire on the following Sunday: 'He would get down later as he is drilling.' This cryptic reference together with a later one referring to his being 'in camp' suggest that he had joined the yeomanry – surprising but not incredible: for his love of riding, his English country-gentleman aspect might have counterbalanced his contempt for all things military which inspired his later escapade, the *Dreadnought* hoax.

Clive and Vanessa were married on February 7, 1907, at St Pancras Register Office and they spent the first part of their honeymoon at Manorbier. Virginia was sufficiently resigned to be able to attend the ceremony without undue distress. They were to be away for three months, though they returned briefly to Gordon Square towards the end of March before leaving for Paris. Adrian and Virginia had moved on March 25. But daunted by the disarray of removal they followed the Bells to Paris on March 28, staying at different hotels but meeting constantly.

It was here that Adrian met Duncan Grant who was to be his lover and lasting friend. He and Virginia were in the Louvre when a young man came up: 'Are you Adrian Stephen? I'm Duncan Grant.' Or so the story goes of their first meeting, Duncan beautiful

[18] Monk's House papers

and engaging with his dark, curly hair and grey-blue eyes, Adrian no less striking when animated, with his classic features, thoughtful blue eyes and fair hair.

Duncan Grant, born in 1885, was the son of a regular soldier, Major Bartle Grant, and spent his early years with his parents in Burma with his father's regiment. During his schooldays he stayed with relatives in England. His aunt, Lady Strachey, persuaded his parents to let him leave St Paul's School and study art at the Westminster School of Art. He was in Italy in 1902–3 and in Paris 1906–7, where he studied under Jacques-Emile Blanche at La Palette. From 1907 he lived increasingly in London, where he met the Bells and their friends, though not, apparently, Virginia and Adrian.

Virginia and Adrian returned to their new home on the south-west corner of Fitzroy Square on April 10. Duncan Grant gives an illuminating account of the house and its occupants: 'On an unforeseen introduction', he writes to a friend, describing Virginia's reaction, 'there was an expression of blazing defiance and a feeling of awkwardness.' A visitor would be shown into Adrian's or Virginia's study, Adrian's on the ground floor, 'his, neat and handsomely lined with books'. Hers, on the floor above, was untidy, books littered all over the floor, her tall desk like a lectern at which she wrote standing up for two hours every day, stood in a good light near the window. The drawing-room on the ground floor was sparsely furnished, with a Dutch portrait of a lady and Leslie Stephen's portrait by G. F. Watts on the walls, and Adrian's pianola.

On June 4 Adrian passed his Finals and was called to the Bar. He began by specialising on wills and probate cases, intriguing subjects for one with his curiosity about the vagaries of human behaviour. Also, he had a feeling for property; he managed the affairs of his family. And when the British Psychoanalytical Society were looking for enlarged premises in 1950, it was Adrian who reported on the suitability of 63 New Cavendish Street, still their premises today.

Virginia entertained a number of guests to tea, friends of their mother's and Stella's – whom Adrian termed 'the Hyde Park Gaters' – as well as her own friends, Violet Dickinson, Madge Vaughan, Lady Eleanor Cecil and Beatrice Thynne. Family friends came, her aunt Caroline Stephen from Cambridge, and her cousin Katherine Stephen. George Duckworth came with his wife (though not often) and Gerald. To complete their household Adrian and Virginia got a dog from the Battersea Dogs' Home. This was Hans, ill-trained, who made the well-documented mess on the carpet when Lady Strachey came, which was ignored by the well-bred ladies and cleared up by Adrian. In the autumn after their return from their summer holiday in Playden, near Rye, Kent, with the Bells near by, Adrian and Virginia resumed the 'Thursday Evenings' begun by Thoby.

> About ten o'clock in the evening people used to appear and continue to come at intervals till twelve o'clock at night, and it was seldom that the last guest left before two or three in the morning. Whisky, buns, and cocoa were the diet. If someone had lit a pipe he would hold out the lighted match to Hans the dog, who snapped at it and put it out. Conversation; that was all. Yet many people made a habit of coming, and few who did will forget these evenings.
>
> Among those who consistently came in the early days were Charles Sanger, Theodore Llewelyn Davies, Desmond MacCarthy, Charles Tennyson, Hilton Young (later Lord Kennet), Lytton Strachey.'[19]

Saxon Sydney-Turner became one of their most frequent visitors, arriving at all hours and often outstaying his welcome. Adrian and Virginia would see him advancing and hide when he tapped on their window. He was one of those strange characters who attach themselves to friends; the link with Adrian was music, particularly opera. Saxon was a serious musicologist; he even 'composed' himself. Virginia complained to a friend about his long sessions at the pianola.

In November 1907, Virginia writes, 'Adrian and I are settled down for the winter. Adrian enjoys his law.' As well as writing for the Cornhill and other literary journalism she was working on *Melymbrosia* which became *The Voyage Out.* She so often writes 'we are settled' that one wonders how much this was wish-fulfilment: she ws determined to make their life together work. Her affection and concern were compounded with guilt. Adrian had his own pre-occupations: his health, for example. In another letter Virginia Woolf mentions his seeing 'a new man', perhaps a urologist? And there was his uncertainty about his growing attraction to Duncan Grant, who had become a frequent visitor. (In November 1909 Duncan took a house, 21 Fitzroy Square, with Maynard Keynes, with whom he had a long-lasting affair.)

[19] *Lytton Strachey*, Vol. 1 by Michael Holroyd

Adrian was companionable enough, a reasonably adequate escort for his sister; they went to the play and to concerts and the opera. They learned German together. And there was frequent intercourse between Gordon Square and Fitzroy Square, the 'Thursday Evenings', Vanessa's Friday Club and a play-reading society, begun on December 21, 1907, alternating between the two houses, with Stephens, Bells, Lytton Strachey, Saxon Sydney-Turner and others. Virginia was frequently absent visiting friends, or on her own, intent on the progress of her novel.

Late in April 1908, she took lodgings in St Ives, and Adrian joined her after a walking tour: 'Adrian came suddenly, that very day, like some grim figure out of a Northern Saga. . . . He had been snowed upon, and hailed upon and rained upon. . . . However, he had had a very good time . . . and had many stories to tell.' There followed a domestic interlude, the Bells arriving with nurse and baby, upon which Adrian left them to have tea in London with Saxon Sydney-Turner and discuss opera. Later on that year she took rooms in Wells, and at Manorbier where she completed the first hundred pages of her novel. She went, too, to Italy and Paris with the Bells. In this way, perhaps, her life with Adrian was made tolerable. She found him 'by turns a depressing and exasperating companion'. Quentin Bell, who knew them both better than anyone now living, writes[20] that Adrian could be

> maddeningly lethargic, lamentably silent, unable to find interest in anything except the constant rehearsal of old family reminiscences . . . he could, on occasion, be gay, enterprising and high-spirited; but such occasions were few and, with his sister, his intelligence and his humour were diverted into a habit of mocking surveillance and quiet irony, a devastating appreciation of other people's faults, and, above all, a merciless vein of pleasantry. Virginia's flightiness brought out his sardonic Stephen matter-of-factness, her enthusiasm his scepticism, her arguments his ridicule. He was a tease and found in Virginia an eminently teasable subject.

Quentin Bell goes on to relate how, when other arguments failed, they threw pats of butter at one another 'so that the walls were starred with flattened projectiles'. There was at least one witness; perhaps it only happened once. Even so, it suggests a kind of

[20] *Biography* of *Virginia Woolf*, Vol. 1, by Quentin Bell.

mutual idiosyncratic craziness, an extreme release of tension. (My first association on reading this was with an occasion in Virginia's life when, much later, Barbara Bagenal was lunching with the Woolfs and Virginia began flicking pieces of meat off her plate. Leonard Woolf motioned to Barbara to stay where she was while he led his wife from the room.)[21]

Clive wrote to Virginia later, in a flirtatious vein, that he had been ashamed at his own cowardice at not sticking up for her when Adrian abused her. Was this more than the usual dismissive brotherly talk about sisters? No doubt he was fond of her in his uncommunicative way, as she was of him. But he seems to have contributed little to their plans and let her take the initiative. It is conceivable that he resented her anxiety about him, her care for him, her treatment of him as 'the poor little boy' of their past family life and their father's crushing references to him in *The Mausoleum Book*. We know he was awed by her as a writer. Some time after the publication of *The Voyage Out* he had to get a friend to tell her how much he had enjoyed it. Perhaps, too, he was awed by her authority as an elder sister.

In August he took off to Bayreuth with Saxon Sydney-Turner. In November Virginia and Adrian stayed with Lytton Strachey at Penmenner House at the Lizard, Cornwall, the small 'town' rather than a village, with houses of granite and the lovely but porous local serpentine, on the very tip of the most southerly peninsula reaching out into the Atlantic. It is a strange bleak place considered as a retreat for Lytton; but it suited his mood, recalling happier days there with G. E. Moore and his 'special congregation of Lytton's Apostolic friends'. After a few peaceful days together spent reading, talking and walking, the Stephens returned home.

Brother and sister spent Christmas 1908, at Fitzroy Square.

[21] In conversation with Mrs Bagenal.

9

ADRIAN'S DIARY

On June 6, 1909 Adrian began to keep a diary. The surviving typescript ends on July 16. If there was more, it has not survived. The story of its discovery by a young bookseller in Cambridge, Massachusetts, is typical of several stories about Adrian, tantalising, tailing away in obfuscation, as though he was covering his tracks. Here is David Garnett's version,[22] written to Olivier Bell on November 2, 1970:

> In, I think, 1923, Mina Kirstein gave a young Cambridge, Mass, bookseller, an introduction to me. He was called Maurice Firuski. Just before we parted he said: 'Have you ever heard of someone called Saxon?' & then told me he had found a treasure – among throw-outs from the Pierpont Morgan Library. He lent me the book written in an exercise book & I showed it to Vanessa. Firuski was contented with a typewritten copy & I kept another & I believe Vanessa returned the original to Adrian. It was surmised that it had been caught up with Thackeray MSS sold to Morgan. There was no more and no other Stephen papers as I know. I think it ought to be published. I am sorry there is nothing more.

Adrian's own version varies slightly but ends in the same frustration. A manuscript had been found, he told me in 1942, speaking as though it had been a recent discovery. His story follows David Garnett's. But when I implored him to let me see it, his teasing reply ended the matter: 'I don't trust you. Besides it's in shorthand.'

When the Diary begins it seems as though Adrian were squaring up to the task of writing it, determined to omit nothing, however

[22] David Garnett in a letter to Olivier Bell, November 2, 1970.

banal. He is at his best when describing friends at dinner and other parties. His observations are acute, though not always kind, specially when he himself is feeling out of sorts. The Diary affords a picture of their life at the time, growing in diversity as he and Virginia expand their acquaintance. Every morning Virginia worked standing at her lectern; and most mornings he worked too in his chambers, though less intensively. He generally lunched at home, occasionally bringing back work. If they weren't going to a concert or a picture gallery, they might stroll about London, go to the Zoo or walk through Kensington Gardens and Hyde Park, staying to listen to the orators at Speakers' Corner, whom Adrian describes in detail – he was as fascinated by the oddity, the quiddity of humankind as Virginia, though she put her interest to better use than he until, nine years later, he trained as a psychiatrist. And there was constant interchange between Fitzroy and Gordon Squares, visits at any hour, separately or together.

During the six weeks covered by the Diary they were a good deal in one another's company, at parties, concerts and the theatre, at dinner parties, and when they entertained at home. On a rare disengaged evening they might dine together, talk a little or sit and read; and Adrian played the pianola with some taste, it may be supposed, for he was as musical as his mother had been and as Virginia was. His diary is full of notes which show his informed critical appreciation of the concerts and operas they heard.

We know something of what Virginia felt about her brother, of how his periodic depression saddened and oppressed her. And she had grief and unhappiness of her own to bear: Thoby's death still darkened both their memories. She became disheartened at the apparent failure of her wish to care for him, to 'make him happy'. Vanessa wrote to a friend, after Virginia had been staying with the Bells in Florence, how sad it was to see her returning home on her own – as though Adrian hardly counted. There may have been, too, the exasperation of his moroseness at home and his only perking up when they went out together or at parties.

The Diary shows that his attitude to her seems typical of that of most men with their sisters – and an elder sister at that. He is critical and dismissive of her and much taken up with his own life. But there are two occasions when his comments on her behaviour go beyond brotherly disapproval. The first, on July 1, at one of their 'Thursday Evenings', is when he describes her cruel treatment of a guest, Annie Cole, abetted by Clive. Under his usual laconic observation one senses that he really minds, both for Virginia and Annie, though he is slow at coming to her rescue. The second occasion is when they were walking in Gordon Square with Clive and Vanessa and Virginia burst into a hysterical tirade of abuse and complaint against them. Why did Adrian find this incident worth recording? And with a changed tone, a departure from his usual laconic, detached chronicle of events? Again one senses that he minds for her, not just for 'making an exhibition of herself', and, on a deeper level, feels compassion for the inner confusion and pain that prompts these exaggerated tirades.

Monday, 7th June
In the morning I made the first entry in my diary. I lunched with Myles, and in the afternoon, having no work to do, I read *The Way of All Flesh*.[23] In the evening Virginia and I went to hear Delius's 'Mass of Life' at the Queen's Hall. It seemed to me to be a dull work and much too long. The last section pleased me more than the others but by the time we reached it I was too much bored to keep my attention properly fixed.

Tuesday, 8th June
After a day spent chiefly on finishing off *The Way of All Flesh*, I went to the Opera . . . Saxon was in the Amphitheatre, when I saw him afterwards pestered me as usual to get him all sorts of tickets, and informed me that though he was going to Drury Lane on Thursday evening he might yet look in upon us later!

Wednesday, 9th June
In the evening Virginia and I called for Vanessa and Clive at Gordon Square and we all went to a party at the Billie Ritchies. The whole place was full of Booths and Ritchies and Meinertzhagens. The thing which struck me most perhaps was the decay of the Booth family; they are none of them very old, but their faces have all fallen in and their cheeks hang in pallid folds about their ugly bones; their voices have dwindled to a mere piping and their minds are shrunk to less than a baby's. The Ritchies on the other hand have swollen, they are blown out like long drowned dogs; Richmond is a mass of corruption.

[23] Samuel Butler's posthumous novel

Wednesday, 16th June
In the evening we gave a dinner party and had as our guests Bruce Richmond, Beatrix [probably Meinertzhagen], Marjorie Strachey and Hawtrey. At table there was a fierce discussion between the last three about the workhouse system, Beatrix making up for lack of information by superiority of lung power; B.R. in the midst of his polite dinner table conversation with Virginia looked round quite astonished by the hubbub, and as soon as he opened his mouth his words were thrust back down his throat by Beatrix, I do not know what he made of it all. When the ladies had gone into the study we talked about Thomas Hardy, Bruce Richmond having a great admiration for him and thinking the Dynasts the greatest work since I don't know when. Later in the evening Vanessa and Clive brought round with them Lady Ottoline and Mr Morell with whom they had been dining and Augustus John and his wife. I heard Clive and Hawtrey and Morell go off upon an appalling political discussion. Marjorie Strachey told peoples characters from their hands, John and Beatrix sat glaring at each other upon the sofa, and I did my best to talk to Lady O. and Mrs John. Lady O. had rather a headache and she and her husband left at about eleven and were followed by Beatrix. Then I engaged Mrs John in conversation about the Opera, simply to have the pleasure of looking at her, as she is one of the most beautiful people I ever saw. She must be partly gypsy I think, and has the most wonderful eyes and thick dark hair; her complexion is perfectly clear and very dark and the shape of her face is exquisite, broad at the cheek bones and coming round to a small chin. She wore a great straw hat which Lady Ottoline gave her and which suits her to perfection. She is obviously the model for many of her husband's pictures. John and she left after he had drunken about half a pint of whiskey and the rest of the party settled down to a good wrangle after the fashion of old Thursday evenings at Gordon Square.

The following description of the fancy-dress ball at the Royal Botanical Gardens (then in the Inner Circle, Regent's Park) shows Adrian at his best, engaged cheerful, observant – and not only of people's ugly defects of character or appearance. His leaning towards the theatre, his unfulfilled wish to choose acting as a career enhanced his love of dressing up. He was a natural mimic, and in costume he became the character he represented. The episode of the ball is a prime example of the energy of youth. They walked home, at three o'clock in the morning, to Bloomsbury. No wonder he was sleepy the following day, though he attended chambers as usual and, hungry after a *nuit blanche*, lunched with two colleagues followed by post-prandial torpor. Finally, that very evening, he and Virginia were off to dine with the Booths. Her reserve of energy is even more impressive than his.

Thursday, 17th June
In the evening we went to dine with Vanessa and Clive before going on to a fancy dress ball at the Botanical Gardens. Virginia after being almost persuaded by Clive to go as a pierette decided to go as Cleopatra; she looked very fine in long flowing robes with her hair down, though more like Isolde than Cleopatra. Vanessa went in a short white satin petticoat tricked out with ribbons and with roses in her hair; very French and improper she looked. Lady Ottoline was dressed in a superb black Spanish costume with a black lace mantilla and was very stately. Morell went in ordinary Court dress. I was in a long red cardinal's robe with a grey wig and skull cap, and Clive was in plain evening dress. There were three huge rooms for dancing and they were all full, but the pleasantest part of the entertainment was sitting out in the Gardens. I danced two or three dances but spent most of the time prowling round examining the various costumes. The only people I really spoke to outside our party were Beatrix and Mary Meinertzhagen with both of whom I sat out. Beatrix Meinertzhagen sat out about three dances running with me and talked about a play she had written and acted at Christmas. We stayed to see the dawn well up and then walked home where we arrived about half past three. It is a great pity that more fancy dress balls are not given. I think they are charming. Of course a very great number of the dresses were purely grotesque but some were really beautiful; Clive indeed, who has been to a large number of these balls, said that it was the finest he had ever seen. I had forgotten to mention that in the afternoon Virginia and I went to a concert at the Queens Hall to hear

Nordica and John Coates sing, with Nikisch conducting the London Symphony Orchestra. Poor Nordica is a fraud, her voice is quite worn out and her singing is too melodramatic for words. . . .

Friday, 18th June
Feeling very sleepy I went out to luncheon with Myles and Vickers; we tried to get in at the Cheshire Cheese but it was full and we went to Simpson's instead. We had a large luncheon of saddle of mutton and beer and then I was more or less torpid till the evening.

Thursday, July 1st
On my way home I went to Gordon Square where I found the Goat and walked home with her. We dined alone together and after dinner waited a long time before anybody appeared. Saxon as usual came in first but was quickly followed by Norton and he by James and Lytton Strachey. We were very silent at first, Virginia and Lytton and I doing all the talking, Saxon being in his usual state of torpor and Norton and James occasionally exchanging a whisper. Later on Vanessa and Clive came in bringing with them Duncan Grant. After this the conversation became more lively. Vanessa sat with Lytton on the sofa and from half heard snatches I gathered they were talking about his and James's obscene loves. Whatever it was they were discussing they were brought to an abrupt stop by a sudden silence, this pleased them very much, especially Vanessa, and I kindly added to their joy by asking why they stopped. Soon afterwards Henry Lamb came in having returned from doing some portraits at Oxford. The conversation kept up a good flow, though it was not very interesting, until at about half past eleven Miss Cole arrived.

She went and sat in the long wicker chair with Virginia and Clive on the floor beside her. Virginia began her usual tone of frank admiration to compliment her on her appearance. 'Of course, you Miss Cole are always dressed so exquisitely. You look so original, so like a sea-shell. There is something so refined about you coming in among our muddy boots and pipe smoke, dressed in your exquisite creations.' Clive chimed in with more heavy compliments and then began asking her why she disliked him so much saying how any other young lady would have been much pleased with all the nice things he had been saying but that she treated him so sharply. At this Virginia interrupted with 'I think Miss Cole has a very strong character' and so on and so on. Altogether Miss Cole was as unhappy and uncomfortable as she could be; it was impossible not to help laughing at the extravagance of Virginia and Clive and all conversation was stopped by their noisy choruses, so the poor woman was the centre of all of our gaze, and did not know what to do with herself. At last, a merciful diversion was made and Virginia took my seat and I hers and with, I may say, some skill I managed to keep Clive under control. James and Lytton Strachey left and we played an absurd game which Vanessa and Clive had learnt at the Freshfields. The principle of the game was as follows: that person won who in half a minute could say the most words beginning with any given letter. Clive held the watch and gave us each our turn. Norton being given G started off with Jerusalem and Jesus which I am afraid must have added another pain to poor Miss Cole's already lengthy list. We all had our turns Vanessa trying to sail as near to the wind as she could, she is always trying to bring out some bawdy remark and is as pleased when she has done it as a spoilt child. Miss Cole went at one and Duncan Grant at about the same time, when a great discussion was started, I know not by whom, about vice. Very soon Virginia with exquisite art made herself the centre of the argument making the vaguest statements with the intensest feeling and ready to snap up anybody who laughed. Her method is ingenious and at first is rather disconcerting for when someone has carefully examined her argument and certainly refuted it she at once agrees with him enthusiastically saying that he has put her point exactly. The argument such as it was degenerated into mere phrasemaking and so regarded was quite amusing; this gave way in its turn to the game of bantering Saxon. He was chaffed and laughed at for all his little peculiarities and all the time he kept his silence only giving an occasional smile. He could not be provoked into saying anything even by Virginia's most daring sallies which never fail of their guffaw when Clive is present. At last everybody went except Saxon. Saxon stayed on to discuss different ways to Germany having obtained further information from Cooks. Virginia and I were however so sleepy that we managed by sheer indifference to oust him. We got to bed just as the dawn was coming up at about 5.

Friday, July 2nd
Virginia and I dined with the Morells before going with them to Don Giovanni. Their house into which I had never penetrated before, is one of the charming Adam houses in Bedford Square, and they have shown considerable taste in its decoration. Only Ottoline and her husband and a Miss Sandys were there. They were full of Henry James who had just been to tea and whom they all worshipped. . . .

Sunday, July 4th
I went to tea at Gordon Square to meet one of George Mallory and James Strachey. James did not appear being busy organising a society for the production of censored plays. Duncan Grant however came in his stead to chaperone Mallory. We talked dully about the play and James Strachey's future – they think he ought to become an actor or a dramatist. George Mallory being 'in love' with him I did not speak out very plainly but thought that he ought to try for a job in a Museum. He seems to have a considerable reputation in Cambridge, though whether he obtains it by silence I don't know. Virginia stayed at home entertaining Lady Gwendolen Godolphin Osborne, a very refined delicate little creature the daughter of the Duke of Leeds. After dinner we both went round to Vanessa and Clive to walk in the Square. We found them already out, and joined them. When we came in Virginia made a violent attack upon them saying how rich they were and how poor she herself was and therefore how much more important it was for her than for them to do work. She became quite virulent so we took to teasing her and at last made her see her ridiculousness. It all arose out of her very transparent fishings for compliments for an article about the Carlyles; Clive and Vanessa had both read it but would not give any criticisms. Clive then, perhaps meanly, but, I think with justification, drew her out with hints of compliments by Norton. Finally we returned home after twelve o'clock.

Thursday, July 8
We had Duncan Grant to dine with us alone. He was very amusing about various parties he had been to lately but I could not reproduce our conversation with any accuracy. Afterwards there came in Lady Ottoline Morell and Mrs Sanger and we had a long discussion about philanthropy. . .

Thursday, July 14
In the evening Mrs MacCarthy dined with us, Desmond having gone to a dinner in honour of Samuel Butler. We, of course, discussed the visit to the Meinertzhagens and she told me she was sure they were Jews, I had always believed it myself until the Booths and others had taken their oaths to the contrary. This would give the impression that our conversation was rather spiteful and unfriendly to the Meinertzhagens but in fact it was quite the reverse. Later Saxon came in and was followed by Vanessa, Duncan Grant and Desmond, and Miss Sheepshanks. We tried to persuade the MacCarthys to take Hyde Park Gate and turn it into a boarding house which should be made a success by Molly's brilliant economy and Desmond's brilliant conversation. I know nothing about the economy, but I really think the conversation would suffice by itself. Desmond was certainly very amusing and altogether I think the evening was very charming.

The Diary, or at least as much of it as we are allowed to see, ends with the entry for Saturday, July 16. Was there more? Or did his increasing though cautious response to Duncan Grant's advances make it impossible for him to maintain his persona adopted in the Diary, that of a young man of good family with taste, judgement, with an informed love of music, and a light-hearted fondness for young women? It was not until 1910 that he openly confessed his love to Vanessa and Virginia.

No doubt the developing situation was observed by friends and family. There is one curious reference in a letter from Virginia to Clive Bell on Christmas Day, 1908. She has been discussing Duncan Grant and goes on: 'Lytton told me the whole story of Adrian's love affair the other day – how he had wept in Boswell's rooms, and yet had never spoken to the man.' The two were such inspired gossips, Virginia so prone to flights of fancy, and the story so much at variance with the facts – we know Adrian met Duncan Grant at least as early as February 1907 – that it would hardly be fruitful to pursue the reference.

On August 5, 1909, Virginia and Adrian set off for Bayreuth, ducking Saxon's usual long discussion as to routes by curtly announcing they were travelling there on their own. On August 9 Adrian writes to Vanessa:

> I suppose that the Goat has described our lodgings already so I only say that she, at any rate, has a very comfortable room. Up to the present moment she and I have been on the best of terms and have even been driven by Saxon's lethargy to fraternise. I need not say that this desirable state of affairs has not been brought about without great forbearance on my part, and I don't know how much longer it will last if she insists on doing any more shopping. I went with her yesterday and bought a pen holder and you know what that means, and then we bought a parasol. She asked for a white one and the woman with exemplary patience brought out every white parasol in the shop & then Virginia said that white ones were no good unless they had green linings; so then she said she would like a coffee coloured one & eventually she bought the cheapest brown holland thing in the shop. When I asked her afterwards why she had asked for a white one when apparently it was the last thing she wanted, she replied that when she said white she only meant that she did not want anything with very bright colours. Later in a bookshop she had all the Tauchnitz editions brought down for her, to see whether they had the Autocrat at the Breakfast Table which had eventually to be sent for from Leipzig; when she got home she found she had packed her own copy after all and wanted to go back & countermand her order; however as I took no notice of her suggestion she subsided; I really could not face the people again. During the journey out Saxon was a little more lively than usual but now signs of mortification are setting in. He is engaged at the moment in writing to Clive and he looks up every now & then to tell me that he has not said anything yet and has got nothing to say so I doubt whether his letter will be very exciting. He has just decided that on the whole he had better use a metaphor. The other night he sang in his sleep;

my room is not entirely partitioned from his and I heard him. His song was a long crackling moaning wail and every now and then he accompanied himself thumping on the bed with his hands.

My travelling companions are a curious pair. I feel like a mad-house keeper.

Yrs,
Adrian Stephen

For God's sake don't tell the Goat anything I have said in this letter. Though she is making great efforts not to be egoistic I am sure she is curious to know what I am telling you.

On August 18 he writes again:

It is a very long time since I wrote to you but I have been so much occupied with going to the opera and looking after my flock that my opportunities have been narrowly limited. I trust I may never have to travel with this pair again, at any rate not to hear music; I am afraid though that this is asking too much of Providence. We must be a curious sight as we leave the opera house between the acts; there is the Goat carrying a parasol, a large leather bag, a packet of cigarettes, a box of chocolates and the libretto in one hand and at the same time vainly striving to hold up a long white cloak & skirt which insist upon trailing in the dust however high she holds them; then there is Saxon humming to himself with an impassioned voice and gesticulating so wildly that one thinks that every bone in his body must be out of joint; then I come holding my head very high & pretending that nothing particular is happening & at the same time trying to lead the others away from the main body of the crowd. It is of no use trying to relieve the Goat of any of her burdens because as soon as one makes the attempt half of them are scattered upon the ground. Eventually I conduct them into a large deserted field when Virginia and I sit down and Saxon also when his rheumatics permit of it; here Saxon always becomes doubly mortish[24] and sour & Virginia begins to expand into the most extravagant images. At last I am driven into contradicting her flatly & she snaps back at me & then we all subside and eat our chocolate in silence and

[24] Adrian's term

> comparative peace. You will see from this that it is not an ideal atmosphere for hearing music and as they have been doing the Ring very badly this cannot be said to be a very merry holiday. I can think of nothing else to say but that Saxon is engaged in cutting a pencil and collecting the chips one by one as they fall, on a little piece of paper which he intends to empty into an ashtray. . . .
>
> yrs Adrian Stephen

Virginia's letters to Vanessa from Bayreuth indicate that she and Adrian are getting on well together, united in opposition to Saxon's eccentricities.

> Saxon can't decide anything – even what he wants to eat – but Adrian is very prompt and businesslike . . . I have been thinking a great deal about father too, and discussing him with Adrian. I believe he was really very modest; he was certainly not self-conscious about his work; nor was he an egoist, as I am. He had very few sympathies though; and practically no imagination . . . Adrian is for the most part, not only clever but even affectionate. For God's sake don't tell him so! This year has made a great difference in him.

On returning Virginia took a cottage near the Bells at Studland, Dorset. Adrian came and stayed. From there she wrote to Violet Dickinson: 'We went to Dresden where we became intimate with an American opera singer who was on the verge of a lawsuit and conferred with Adrian every afternoon in her bedroom.' This must be the explanation of an incident told by the family and confirmed by his daughter Ann. Adrian went to Chattanooga, Tennessee, settled her affairs and returned home three days later – an incident which shows the impulsive, quixotic side of his nature. He would go to some length to help anyone in distress, particularly if it involved an adventure.

On Christmas Day 1909, Virginia wrote to Vanessa from Lelant in Cornwall: 'Lytton came and we were very intimate and easy. . . . But Duncan Grant also arrived, which was a little difficult. He went in ten minutes.'

This suggests that Adrian's affair with Duncan was progressing. Maynard Keynes was deeply hurt by this new love. In November

1909 he moved from St James's Court to 21 Fitzroy Square where Duncan had a studio at the front of the house, Maynard an inadequate room at the back. His behaviour was as wise as it was generous. He realised that he could not prevent this new serious love; but by keeping Duncan's friendship he could remain his protector. In two restrained, truthful letters exchanged on the December 18 and 19, Keynes and Duncan Grant defined their relationship:

Dearest Duncan
It makes me miserable not to find you here – though I expected that you would in the end stay at 29. I don't know what to do about staying in London. You're married to Adrian now, which you weren't before. So you naturally want always to be with him, when you haven't got any necessary engagements. So I will hardly ever see you except when out of kindness you think you ought to try and make some arrangements. Thus I'm always in the position of pressing you to do what you'd rather not, and you of wondering how much your fondness for me demands of you. I can't bear such a state of affairs. It's wretched to be trading on your kindness, and I'm always in a state of uncertainty as to whether you will in the end turn up.

What do you think? It seems to me that when you are alone with me it's all right. But when Adrian is in the next house, whenever you're with me it's being away from him, and you see me because I want it, not because you do. Please don't misunderstand this letter. It's the fault of fate and not at all of yours. But I'm feeling very wretched and don't know what I ought to do. Your ever loving,

JMK

PS. Please when you read this letter try and decide exactly what [. . .]

Dearest Maynard,
Please do not be so depressed. I hope most of your depression is the result of severe tiredness and overwork, because I don't honestly think things have changed as much as you think. I certainly am not always wishing to be with Adrian

when I am with you. For one thing it is not always possible to be with him & when I am as certain as I am of Adrian's affection for me, I can afford to be much 'kinder' as you call it than the case when I was uncertain about it. I simply mean that I have none of the anxieties that I used to have & can therefore enjoy myself in every way more than I used to including being with people I like.

To be quite practical I should probably be in the studio in any case . . . for nearly all day every day. I might want to be with Adrian in the evening but there do occur occasions when I cannot. I don't know how you would like this state of affairs – but it would mean seeing you a good deal. . .

Yrs, Duncan Grant

10

THE DREADNOUGHT HOAX

'From time to time . . . there has arisen a queer stir of interest in what was once called "The Dreadnought Hoax".' Thus Adrian begins his true story,[25] told in spare, convincing prose, of the most audacious, elaborate, unlikely deception ever perpetrated. The sequel to the Cambridge hoax, carried out in 1905, was more ambitious: nothing less than holding up to ridicule the Royal Navy, then at the height of its majesty, determined to keep its dominance in the face of Kaiser Wilhelm's ambition to make Germany a great sea power. Adrian relates how the plan was first suggested to Cole by a naval officer who wanted to pull another officer's leg. This appealed to Adrian because the officer's intended victim was one of his own Fisher cousins, chief of staff to the admiral of 'the Channel Fleet' (as Adrian believed it was called), then lying at Weymouth. The flagship was HMS *Dreadnought*, the last word in battleship construction. They proposed to visit it in the character of the Emperor of Abyssinia and his suite.

This preposterous plan was worked out over luncheon and put into action without delay. Cole was to be a young gentleman from the Foreign Office, Anthony Buxton, a Cambridge friend, was cast as the Emperor, Guy Ridley, an Oxford man, Duncan Grant and Adrian's sister Virginia (roped in at the last minute to augment the suite, in spite of the appalled remonstrance of Vanessa). Adrian, lightly disguised in a false beard, a moustache and a dusting of sunburn powder, was the Foreign Office interpreter. Wearing a greatcoat and carrying an umbrella, he looked like 'a seedy commercial traveller'. With his great height, disguise in the event of his meeting an acquaintance was almost impossible. The others were suitably dressed and made up by Clarkson's, the well-known theatrical cos-

[25] *The Dreadnought Hoax*, Hogarth Press, 1936; new edition with introduction by Quentin Bell, 1983.

tumiers, and the great Willy Clarkson himself came to Gordon Square to superintend though 'of course we let no one into the plot'. With typical Stephen aplomb a telegram signed 'Hardinge' (the permanent head of the Foreign Office) was despatched to the Admiral; and on February 10 the hoaxers entrained at Paddington for Weymouth.[26] Adrian and Cole lunched in the dining-car – lunch there was forbidden to the others 'as we were afraid of accidents to their make-up'. During their meal Cole, aided by a grammar bought from the Society for the Propagation of the Gospel, attempted to teach Adrian some elementary Swahili which, they believed, was spoken in some parts of East Africa. 'Of course I could hardly remember two words though some newspapers described us as having spoken "fluent Abyssinian".' But it helped to pass the time for 'to tell the truth we were feeling rather nervous. Something so easily might go wrong. It might be that the telegram ought to have been written in some special code . . . or perhaps my cousin might recognise me.' But Adrian was a gambler, a poker player, never cooler than when involved in some hazardous situation. 'I think that perhaps the most exciting moment was first the arrival at Weymouth – that was the plunge into the cold bath. As the train slowed down for the station we were all agog. I think I half-expected that no notice would be taken of us at all, and we should have to slink back to London, but, no, there on the platform stood a naval officer in full uniform and the hoax had begun.'

A red carpet had been laid on the platform, a barrier erected to keep sightseers at a respectful distance; and the party were driven to the harbour where a steam launch awaited them. By this time the expedition had become 'almost an affair of every day . . . It was hardly a question any longer of a hoax. We were almost acting the truth. Everyone was expecting us to act as the Emperor and his suite.' As they steamed alongside, the pride of the Royal Navy seemed smaller and uglier than he had expected. However, he 'had not much time for criticism' for the Admiral and his staff and the captain of the *Dreadnought* were ready to receive them. Adrian boarded last and was taken aback when Cole, who was introducing the party, referred to him as 'Kauffman', not the English name he had chosen but Cole had misheard. Adrian was 'a little alarmed because German spy scares were for ever being started in those days . . . At the same time I was conscious of looking the most awful "outsider", not knowing whether to take my hat off or shake hands.' Other causes for alarm were his noticing that his cousin (the naval

[26] Then a Great Western Railway station.

officer) was staring at him and the discovery that the ship's captain himself was an acquaintance. However, 'I was saved by the naval officers' proverbial tact. Their cordiality was such that it put me at my ease at once.' And the inspection of the ship proceeded.

Translating English into Abyssinian presented some difficulty as the few Swahili words he had learned in the train soon ran out, but on the assumption that few naval officers were classicists, he reeled off passages from Virgil and Homer that he had learned by heart at school. As an extra precaution Adrian changed his 'rather high register and Cambridge accent' to 'a most unnatural deep bass, and an accent that was meant to be German'.

The guard of honour inspected, the Admiral handed the party over to the ship's captain, and they were taken on a tour of the ship – the wireless room, the Mess and a demonstration of the guns being turned in all directions. All this Adrian passed on to the Emperor in a mixture of Virgil and Homer. In case hospitality would damage their make-up he declined the invitation to partake of food and drink, explaining that religious beliefs made it impossible for the Royal Family to touch food unless it was prepared in special ways. That dealt with, he had a bad moment when he saw Duncan Grant's moustache beginning to peel off. A light rain had begun to fall. He did what he could with an umbrella but there were five people to cover so he requested that the party should go below to shelter from the chilly weather of England.

Before they re-embarked on the launch Adrian was consulted about the firing of guns to salute the Emperor. With his natural consideration for the crew who would have had to clean the guns, and with his instinctive diplomacy, he told the officer a salute was not necessary: 'The French had not saluted us at Toulon, why should the English?' Another young officer explained that the ship's bandmaster had not been able to find a copy of the Abyssinian national anthem but played, as the next best thing, the anthem of Zanzibar. This, thought Adrian, did excellently, remembering Cole's and his own earlier escapade! There were no further incidents of note beyond Cole trying to pin a fancy-dress order on the breast of a young officer[27] in command of the launch (which he shyly refused as he could not accept it without permission from his superiors) and tipping the crew 'royally'.

When they settled down in the train, all, except Cole, were exhausted and they 'only kept up the hoax so far as to insist on the waiters in the restaurant car wearing white gloves'. That might have

[27] 'He was a nice young man and I was really saddened a few years later when I saw what I believed to be his name in the list of those killed in battle.'

been the end of the affair but Cole could not resist leaking the story to the press. Several weeks later Adrian's naval cousin called wanting them all to apologise. Adrian did not mind apologising in the least if 'it would make things easier for the Admiral' – there had been questions asked in the House of Commons; but he could not answer for the others. Then, 'innocent as a lamb', he gave him their names. He had been hoaxed in his turn for the names were needed for another purpose! The honour of the Royal Navy had been besmirched; the Admiral had been unable to go ashore without having 'Bunga-Bunga' shouted after him, a phrase alleged by the press to have been used by the hoaxers. 'Naturally I was very sorry about this – we had no wish to make anyone really uncomfortable.' To save the Admiral further embarrassment Adrian and Duncan called, unannounced, on the First Lord of the Admiralty, Mr McKenna. As Adrian remarks, 'Perhaps he was laughing up his sleeve.' But he received them assuming that 'we had come to beg for mercy'. At least one of the hoaxers, he said, had committed a forgery over the telegram and was liable to go to gaol under the Post Office Act. 'I think I felt quite ill-used over this. We had come absolutely gratuitously to make what seemed a generous offer.' Perhaps Mr McKenna did not know how to act; the interview ended and Adrian and Duncan were 'bundled out' of his office. Meanwhile Adrian's cousin and another officer called on Cole and announced that they had come to avenge the Navy and proposed to thrash him. But he had just recovered from a serious illness and this put them in a dilemma. Cole suggested that he would agree to be beaten if he was allowed to reply in kind. Six ceremonial taps were applied to his hindquarters and he reciprocated likewise.

Duncan Grant was less fortunate. He was called on while breakfasting with his parents, tripped up and bundled into a taxi which drove off to, according to Virginia Woolf, Hampstead Heath, where he was told to get out. He put up no resistance. 'I can't make this chap out,' said one of the officers, 'he does not put up a fight. You can't cane a chap like that.' In the end Duncan received two taps, also ceremonial ones, and the little party broke up. Why Adrian was not approached he never understood.

So the *Dreadnought* hoax ended. The officers had had their revenge. Adrian concluded his history as follows: 'They treated us so delightfully while we were on board that I, for one, felt very uncomfortable at mocking, even in the friendliest spirit, such charming people.' There is a postscript to the story quoted in

Geoffrey Maddan's Notebooks[28] which would have amused the participants. Two young midshipmen were heard conversing during the inspection of the ship: 'You haven't been in the East – they've got the real nigger smell.' The source of this anecdote is attributed to Dr George Rylands, who can't remember the quotation but has allowed me to use it.

From March 10 onwards, Virginia's health was precarious. It is questionable whether Adrian was wise to persuade her, against Vanessa's opposition, to take part in the drama and uncertainty of the *Dreadnought* hoax. After a short visit with the Bells to Lelant in Cornwall she was ill in bed. On March 26 they took her to Studland Bay in Dorset for three weeks' rest, where Adrian joined them. It was there that Vanessa wrote to Lytton Strachey that he seemed more than usually depressed and withdrawn. 'He has been sunk in gloom ever since he arrived . . . literally sitting in an armchair all Saturday, Sunday and today, except for two short walks of at most half-an-hour each. He doesn't even read, and I can't imagine why he's come.'

He was, one can only guess, tormented by uncertainty, and perhaps shame, about his affair with Duncan Grant, overwhelmed by the strength of a passion he had never before experienced. He may also have been affected by the aftermath of his venereal disease, in spite of medical reassurance that no genital symptoms persisted after the first three months.

On May 17 Adrian wrote a letter to Duncan Grant typical of the cautious side of his nature. Whatever physical expression of their friendship had occurred during their three years' friendship the letter marks a definitive advance.

> I had half expected a letter from you this morning as I had thought of writing to you myself, but I was a little surprised at the contents of the letter when it came. The surprise was pleasant, for I had expected abuse, but you cannot hide it from me that I have treated you rather badly. I hope that in future I shall be more careful. I have been thinking over our relations & I will tell you tomorrow what conclusions I have reached. In the meantime let me say this, that I am very fond of you indeed & that I see no chance of ceasing to be so & that I shall be very unhappy if you ceased to care for

[28] Edited by J. A. Gere and John Sparrow, Oxford Paperback.

me. I shall expect you at tea tomorrow.

Duncan, then, came to tea next day. Adrian had made up his mind to yield unreservedly to his own passionate feeling. To know that he loved and was loved – was he ever again to experience that first timeless joy of their embrace, oblivious of past or future?

For Duncan, as Adrian already knew, led a complicated emotional life; it is not enough to say he was promiscuous, though he was; sex and friendship between several lovers at once coexisted and some lasted for years. He was beautiful, intelligent, talented, desired by both sexes. When asked to describe him, a young woman of a later generation replied, smiling happily, 'He was a charmer', as though that said everything. Karin Costelloe (who was later to marry Adrian) knew him in Paris. She was not, she writes in her diary, exactly in love with him; she hoped to win his friendship if only she did not talk too much or embarrass him with too many personal questions. He was, she observed, curiously innocent.

He was truly sorry when he turned out to have hurt one of his lovers, as his letters make clear. As early as 1905, when he was seventeen, he wrote to Lytton from Paris, 'I am afraid this letter will give you a great deal of worry and pain perhaps . . . but it is better, far better, that you should read this before you see me again though it makes me miserable to write.' Six years later it is Lytton's younger brother James who is in love with him. Duncan writes to Lytton, 'I'm afraid it was an awful letter . . . but it was frightfully difficult to say anything.'

Adrian, therefore, had to accept that he would always have to share Duncan's love. But in June he felt sufficiently secure to talk to Vanessa. Even then his reticence prevented him from speaking plainly; he talked of 'inversion' in an evasive manner as though ignoring the fact that his affair was common knowledge.

By this time Vanessa was seriously disturbed about Virginia's health. She consulted Dr Savage and others, and at length persuaded Virginia to go into a nursing home in Twickenham run by a Miss Thomas, who was to become Virginia's devoted friend.

Virginia had been finding life with Adrian increasingly unsatisfactory. His habitual moodiness was worsened by uncertainty over his affair with Duncan Grant. Any emotional commitment with men or women tended to throw him into depressed apathy; and there was the additional burden of having to recognise his own capacity for a homosexual relationship. On the other hand Duncan, for whom love came so easily, so simply, offered Adrian what he most needed, the certainty of being loved, the relief of surrendering wholly to the fulfilment of desire.

His inner turmoil bore heavily upon Virginia. Their companionship, Adrian's willing compliance as an escort to concerts, parties, dinner parties, sharing in their success as party-givers, those lighthearted walks in the park, teas and ices at Rumpelmayer's – all that was more or less over by the end of 1909. It must be said that his ironic comments on his sister in correspondence and in his diary contrast sharply with her generous, affectionate references to him in her letters. In fact, during the difficult period after 1906, the loss of Thoby and Vanessa's marriage, Virginia, for all her knife-edge frailty of mind, behaved with admirable sense and stability.

She it was who found 38 Fitzroy Square. Now, half-way through 1910, since they could not live happily together, she outlined a plan to find a bigger house suitable for them to set up a communal ménage shared with chosen friends, to which Adrian willingly assented, without being foremost in searching for the new home.

Small wonder that, with her own social life, her own friendships to enlarge in the face of her extreme diffidence and multiple anxieties, above all her overriding need for peace and continuity in working on her novel, *Melymbrosia*, she should have come near to total breakdown.

Towards the beginning of August 1910, Adrian took rooms in Ingoldswell, a village near Skegness in Lincolnshire, where he stayed for some six weeks. Why did he choose, at this crisis in his life, to cut himself off, to decamp to this unfamiliar, beautiful countryside with its vast curving bay, sandy shores and unbroken skyline? Perhaps because he hoped for privacy in love-making with Duncan. Or because he needed time to accustom himself to this new turn in his life – almost as though he was running away. It may also be that he was uncertain about his health; and still anxious about the possible though unlikely residual symptoms of his venereal disease. (On his return to London he consulted a doctor.)

On August 16 he wrote to Duncan that he had booked a room for him at the weekend. 'When you come, I suppose I may find out the real reason why you did not come last Saturday.' He offers for his distraction some boy scouts encamped near by: 'They don't appeal to me much but you will probably like at least to watch them bathing.'

On August 31 he wrote again, 'You are to come not a moment later than Saturday & I shall beat you if you don't.'

All August saw Adrian slipping and sliding on the sandhills, playing cricket with the little boys, running barefoot along the ribbed sea-sand, ricking his ankle, passing the time of day with the other visitors. In late September they were all gone. Shops selling buckets and spades and shrimping nets were putting up the shutters; the village was turning in on itself in readiness for the long, cold winter. The nip of late autumn was in the Lincolnshire air and can be felt in the next letter to Duncan on September 20. He was more than usually anxious about Duncan's activities, and wretchedly jealous.

> What terrifies me now is that after your 4½ hours conversation with Keynes you will think me such a dullard, if you think of me at all, that you won't think me worth writing to. I hate Keynes for this reason and also for the news you sent me on the postcard. Was ever such news sent on a postcard before? In my cooler moments I can see that it would be absurd of me to raise any objections, but you do make me very jealous indeed. On the whole I think it would be bad luck on poor Keynes to deny him his pleasure and it would not do any good to anyone else. . . . I wish now that I had been content to wait and have you in the second part of September; you would be here now. But perhaps you could never have torn yourself from Keynes' arms. . . . I expect to go back to London on October the first and I shall be quite alone for some time; it is brutish of me but I still hope you will be there for some part of this time too. You appear to be getting too much attracted by Keynes' sister and I am jealous of her as well. . . . Your loving Adrian Stephen.
>
> P.S. The sign on my last letter you misread. It was a conventionalised mouth and was intended to express my desire to kiss you.

Back in London, Adrian seems brighter, more positive. On October 4 he wrote:

My own dearest Duncan
Please don't be jealous about me. There is no one in the world whom I care for half as much as I do for you. . . . It is so hard to explain one's feelings in writing but I shall be seeing you almost as soon, if not before, you get this letter. I don't think there is really any need for anxiety and I am feeling perfectly well. . . . I have just been having an interview with Vinogradoff[29] who has given me a lot of photographs of Manuscripts which I have to decipher and translate for the seminar. . . . You are absurdly kind to insist on having any affection for me after the way in which I treat you. Your loving Adrian Stephen.

[29] Sir Paul Gavrilovitch Vinogradoff, 1854–1925, legal historian. Left Russia in 1902 in protest at Tsarist Government interference in university appointments, appointed Professor of Roman Law at Oxford.

11

THE NEO-PAGANS

During 1911, Virginia and Adrian saw less and less of one another. Virginia spent much of her time at Firle, furnishing 'Little Talland House', as her new home was called, and inviting friends to stay. For his part, Adrian was almost entirely preoccupied with his love for Duncan, though he still continued to work for 'Vino', collating, transcribing and translating medieval Latin manuscripts.

Before Duncan's departure abroad in March he and Adrian went to a Post-Impressionist ball with Roger Fry, Vanessa, Virginia and Clive Bell. The theme was inspired by Gauguin's South Sea Islands paintings, and the women scandalised press and public by their scanty attire. David Garnett gives an account of a similar occasion in *The Golden Echo,*[30] differing as to place and time but with a memorable description of Adrian.

> Brynhild came by flashing a bewitching smile, and Maitland departed in her wake. The Oliviers were there, Godwin Baynes, the Thorneycrofts – and then I noticed a strange, tall figure, made taller still by the very tall hat of a Persian Magus and long oriental robes. Altogether he, with his hat, must have been nearly seven feet high. He had hollow lantern jaws and a slightly bewildered air of astonished amusement. I went up to him at once and hailed him with delight, without the shyness I felt for more ordinary persons. It was Adrian Stephen, whom I had met once before and knew from the first moment of meeting that we were friends.
>
> Adrian had extraordinarily innocent eyes: he looked through them at the passing scene like the child in Hans Christian Andersen's story of the Emperor's New Clothes – as though he could not believe what he saw. Then, aware of

[30] 1953

the inadequacy of words, he caught one's eye and either made a most horrific comic grimace, or laughed.

In March and April Maynard Keynes and Duncan travelled in Greece – they too, like the Stephen brothers in 1906, explored the Peloponnesus, mostly riding. From there they went to Tunis for a few days then crossed to Sicily, Taormina, Syracuse and Palermo. But their plans were curtailed by Adrian's letters proposing that Duncan and he should meet in Naples. (He had invented nick-names for them: Duncan was 'Bear', he was 'Corby' or the Crow.) He planned to reach Naples on Saturday, April 8 at 2.00 p.m.

> I hope that the old bear will arrive there as soon as possible afterwards and not be led astray by the monster Keynes whom I do not trust at all. . . . As soon as the old crow arrives he will fly to the topmost point of Vesuvius[31] and watch steadfastly for the beast's form crossing the plain beneath. It will be fun being together almost worth the separation – we have never been alone together for a fort-night in our lives. Do take care of yourself old beast.
>
> Tonight the Goat and the crow are going to hear Richter conduct the London Symphony Orchestra for the last time.
>
> Good bye your loving Adrian Stephen.

On March 30 he wrote from Fitzroy Square, 'My Darling Bear, This letter is primarily about plans. I am going to be abominably selfish as usual and I can only pray for your forgiveness. I am going to get a return ticket from Marseilles . . . I do not want to force your hand in any way but if you could face the journey back by sea with me I should be only too anxious to pay any extra expense.'

Adrian's letters continued even while he travelled towards his beloved. They flew before him like carrier pigeons, from snow-bound Firle, in the train to Paris after a rough crossing, one from Paris, another in the train to Marseilles, even one from Marseilles as he embarked for Naples.

Neither Adrian nor Duncan comes well out of this permutation of their eternal triangle. Maynard Keynes, who followed Duncan to Naples, wrote reproaching him for being unfeeling: 'Dearest Duncan, I came deeply needing some open sign of affection, and though I felt you had some affection for me underneath, you

[31] A drawing is inserted of a crow poised on a crag watching a bear below.

seemed sodden and had none to give away to me.'[32]

Adrian's meeting with Ray Costelloe was at Little Talland House where he was storm-bound, waiting to cross the channel. 'I liked her,' he wrote to Duncan. Ray was to become his sister-in-law. Virginia had met Ray and Karin Costelloe in October 1910 when she visited their uncle, Logan Pearsall Smith and his sister Alys Russell, called by the girls 'Aunt Lou', at Iffley near Oxford. Virginia had taken to Ray and invited her to Little Talland House. She revisited them in January 1911 when she met Katherine Cox, Rupert Brooke's lover. As before, it was Virginia who broke new ground, Adrian who followed.

The Brookes and the Stephens had been family acquaintances, and Rupert, an 'Apostle', had links with Lytton Strachey and a slightly older generation. Rupert and Ka Cox introduced Virginia to a circle of young people whose style was rather different from that of her Bloomsbury background. Most of the girls were from Newnham, a few of the men had been Bedalians. They enjoyed open-air life, camping, bathing together naked, all with what Quentin Bell has described as 'a sort of innocent camaraderie'. They were what my grandmother would have called 'wholesome'. Virginia herself, while staying with Rupert at Grantchester, bathed naked with him at night in the river, an incident which led Adrian to refer, unkindly and inappropriately, to 'Rupert's Romance'. The Neo-Pagans, as they came to be called, were among the first of their kind to make friendship between the sexes possible without immediate sexual confrontation.

When Rupert Brooke daringly organised the first Bloomsbury Neo-Pagan camp in Devon, Virginia and Maynard Keynes survived the Spartan ordeal best: James Strachey retreated after one night under the stars (there were no tents), and accommodation had already been found for Lytton at a nearby guesthouse. Not for another year did Adrian repeat their experiment.

Among the Neo-Pagans who most appealed to Virginia were the Olivier girls, Margery, Brynhild, Daphne and Noel.[33] Socially their background was similar to the Stephens' but their upbringing was very different: their father, Sir Sydney Olivier, a Fabian Socialist, had entered the Colonial Office the better to foster his aims. Their house at Limpsfield, Chart, was in one of the wilder parts of Surrey on the North Downs, near David Garnett who grew up with them. They were all intelligent, attractive and clever, Brynhild the most

[32] *John Maynard Keynes* by Robert Skidelsky.

[33] *Neo-Pagans* by Paul Delaney.

strikingly beautiful, Daphne hardly less so. But it was Noel, the youngest, who attracted the most attention and most interested Virginia. When Noel was only fifteen Rupert Brooke, who was twenty, fell in love with her. By 1912, when she was nineteen, three men at least were 'chasing' her: Bécassy, a Hungarian Bedalian, James Strachey – and Adrian Stephen.

Adrian's last letter to Duncan from 29 Fitzroy Square is not dated but was probably written early in July 1911. He has consulted Dr MacDonald.[34] On a further visit his doctor is on holiday so he is unable to have blood tests. (These presumably were monitoring the presence of spirochetes in the blood.) He assures Duncan that he is 'all right', that he really isn't unwell. It may be that his heart was affected – the most usual sequel to the infection he had contracted in 1907. Yet he was a prodigious walker in all weathers. In the same letter he writes that Leonard Woolf, on leave after seven years as a colonial servant in Ceylon, had come to tea.

> I liked him very much, what I saw of him. He seems very like what he was at Cambridge except that he has become rather mellower and he was very amusing about Ceylon. His descriptions of hanging were very interesting. . . . He went away to dine with Saxon but said he was going afterwards to the Sangers and would call here to see whether we would come too. Virginia had got tickets for a promenade concert but we arranged to leave it early and get back here in time to meet him. It was too funny, after coming in she went up deliberately and changed her costume in spite of the fact that it was pelting with rain put on her best Turkish cloak and satin slippers and so on. Saxon, Woolf and I were kept waiting while she did all this and then we had to take a taxi. She made great eyes at Woolf whom she called markedly Leonard which seems to be a little forward. Her method of wooing is to talk about nothing but fucking and [illegible] which she calls with a great leer copulation and WCs and I dare say she will be successful, I hope so anyway. . . . It suddenly strikes me that you may think some of the things I have said in my letter unkind. I hope you won't think any the worse of me for them. . . . The Goat sends her love. . . . Write and tell me all that happens to you dear old beast and don't be hard on me. Your loving Crow.

[34] Then a senior house surgeon at St Peter's Hospital for Stone and Urinary Diseases.

By October Adrian and Virginia had chosen a house for their communal ménage on the north side of Brunswick Square. They moved in towards the end of November. Virginia ceaselessly energetic, had also found another house near Firle in Sussex. On November 20 she and Adrian took up their new life at Brunswick Square, with Maynard Keynes, Duncan Grant and, in December, Leonard Woolf.

Life in the ménage suited Adrian. He was among friends for whom he had no responsibility except to see that they paid their monthly share of the outgoings. Their lives went on around him so that he need not feel isolated, yet he could be private in his own quarters. He gave poker parties in the big drawing-room on the first floor, with one wall decorated by a large fresco by Duncan and Adrian, of a mixed tennis doubles, in Post-Impressionist style. As he sat at the table, shuffling and dealing the cards, smoking his pipe with whisky at his elbow, his expression gave way to a relaxed contentment that belied his intense concentration on the game.

One younger friend whom he liked and took up was David Garnett who frequently attended his parties, and felt that 'Adrian's house in Brunswick Square was my spiritual home and his friends . . . were the people I should most like to know. I liked the way they sat about, the way they talked, the entirely casual way in which one of them . . . would fill up his tumbler with Adrian's whisky, without being asked, and others just shook their heads if offered it, without bothering to say thank you.'[35]

As the evening wore on other people would come in after dinner parties or the opera, Ray and Karin Costelloe, Vanessa and Clive, Virginia and Leonard Woolf and Duncan Grant, who for some reason did not care for David Garnett or 'Bunny' as he was called. Nevertheless Adrian continued to invite him. Adrian David found unpredictable:

> He was always unexpected. One night we stayed playing late and did not break up till two o'clock in the morning. The Piccadilly tube would be shut; I should have to walk home to Kensington, for though I had been winning, I should never at that time have taken a cab for myself, even if I had had ten pounds in my pocket.
>
> 'Let's go to the races,' said Adrian as we got up from the table. Gerald Shove and Clive greeted the suggestion with enthusiasm. Maynard was more cautious.

[35] *The Golden Echo*

'What races?' he asked.

'There are sure to be races somewhere,' said Adrian, and as we went out into that clear odd light there is in London in the very early hours of a June morning, Adrian called out to a passing cab:

'Will you drive us to the races, cabby?'

The taxi-man drew up and looked at us curiously. We were not bookies or ordinary race goers and he was puzzled and for a moment or two seemed lost in thought.

'We could make it all right, but it's a long way.'

'Where are they?' asked Maynard.

'Pontefract,' replied the cabby, 'in the West Riding.'

Even Adrian's casual enthusiasm was put off by the notion of a two-hundred mile taxi-drive and amidst general laughter the project was postponed for another occasion.[36]

By 1912 the tone of Adrian's letters to Duncan Grant began to alter. His obsession is gradually loosening its hold, mutating into the friendship that was to last for a lifetime. He had met the Olivier girls and has taken Daphne to a concert. There is mention of an actress called 'Shelley'; on one of his gallant, impulsive missions on behalf of women in trouble he had been to Paris to bring her back to England. 'The poor creature is in love with Cole[37] who treats her shockingly.'

He still 'confesses his sins' to Duncan, describing in detail his visits to prostitutes, even the most ordinary masturbation, though whether his 'sins' are disloyal to Duncan or an offence against the conventional code of his time is not clear.

Adrian's natural bent was heterosexual. As far as is known Duncan was his only homosexual lover. In Duncan's absence he was in need not just of sexual relief but of womanly comfort which the 'Jessie Tanners' and the 'Mrs Walters' gave him. When Duncan was there he provided both. But the complex burden of Adrian's guilt prevented him from the full enjoyment of either. His early guilt arising from his mother's death, his unconscious anger at her broken trust and her desertion were at the root of his adult insecurity – betraying anxiety and jealousy, as when Duncan left him during their holiday at Skegness. And his childhood trauma was accentuated by Thoby's death, compounded by family and friends: 'The wrong man died.' Added to this was the legacy of his parents'

[36] Ibid

[37] Not Horace Cole. Probably Molar Cole who consulted Adrian professionally.

upbringing in the Evangelical sect and their conversion to agnosticism. There is no stricter adherent to moral principles, no more anxious searcher of his or her conscience than a converted agnostic.

From Asheham in April (or later) he wrote to Duncan: 'We have bashed a good deal up in the half-made terrace . . . Darling old thing, there is nothing to report. . . . No letter from Noel.' In an undated note written from Brunswick Square Adrian wrote briefly: 'Darling old beast, hadn't you better go down to Asheham for the weekend. It is so beastly alone here. If you like to stay there until Wednesday and come up with Clive and Nessa I will do your move for you. It won't be very difficult. Anyhow I think it will be better if you went off for the weekend. Love Corby.'

This rather peremptory casual note suggests an increase in Adrian's independence. It is clear from Virginia's letters and from the talk among her circle that he was already openly in love with Noel Olivier, the usual inhibitions preventing him from being at his best. He became, Leonard wrote to David Garnett, 'still more lethargic, inert and depressed, and aloof when rejected by her'.[38] Noel for her part seems to have been repelled by him.

Backed up by Duncan, Adrian went down to Surrey where they found the elder Oliviers playing tennis while their juniors, David Garnett and Noel, retrieved tennis balls. Adrian went off for a walk with Noel, while Duncan detained 'Bunny'. Afterwards she wrote to Rupert Brooke: 'I tried to be reasonable and wrote a confused letter to that Adrian, a blunt thing, mostly a muddle and I *can't* tell whether it will do him any good, or whether it's an awful mistake; it's so difficult to do the right thing in cold blood, I almost thought I oughtn't to meddle with him at all, with my silly *sorryness* and absurd pity, I ought simply to hate him passionately, and let that direct the whole thing, these wise reasonings are insane.'[39]

Rupert Brooke had rightly suggested that it was a kind of game, Adrian's true feelings masked by confusing and distasteful velleities. Yet he was, or longed to be, deeply serious. Years later he told me that Noel was the woman he would most liked to have married. (He thought of love between the sexes in terms of marriage.) He had before him the ideal of a family, of re-creating that lost family so often in mind. (His frequent reminiscences bored his sisters beyond endurance.) Yet, as will be seen, it was that very past which came between him and choosing a woman who could fulfil his ideal. He

[38] *The Letters of Leonard Woolf*, ed. Frederic Spotts.
[39] *The Neo-Pagans* by Paul Delaney.

and his father were alike in some respects: they were both uxorious. But Sir Leslie, unlike his son, twice chose women who could satisfy his needs.

For nearly two years Adrian, bitterly unhappy at his rejection, mourned for Noel. She, for her part, seems to have moderated her ire against him. On a visit to Asheham she found that he, too, had been invited. She was furious. (Virginia, Vanessa noted, had been 'buttering up' Noel in an attempt to elicit a favourable response to her brother's advances. But 'she won't succeed', Vanessa rightly guessed.)

'All the time', Noel writes to Rupert Brooke, 'I worked up an odious indignation against the good Adrian; not even to be calmed by his radiant beauty, as it appeared when he dined in his pyjamas (though it touched me considerably, my hatred only subsided after I had left him, in Bloomsbury on a Monday morning. . .). Later on I felt much more amiable.'

In August 1913, at a camp at Brandon in Norfolk, organised by Vanessa, Adrian photographed the party. There is Noel in the background, a kerchief round her head, doing something useful; Maynard Keynes sprawling in his tent reading the newspaper, Vanessa and Duncan Grant painting at their easels, more Olivier girls and Bloomsbury friends, Roger Fry, Clive Bell and Molly MacCarthy. Adrian seems to have accepted the situation; he occupied himself by work for Vinogradoff and travelling with Duncan in Italy, ending in Paris where Duncan had an invitation to visit Matisse. He spent some time in Germany improving his German and going to the opera. Virginia was married in May 1912, but he was absent. Why? Other relations and friends were there.

In August 1912, he wrote to her from Munich where he, Marjorie and James Strachey were *en pension* at Frau Knoldt's, Nikolai Platz:

> My dear Goat
> I am afraid that I have been rather bad about letter writing but there has been absolutely nothing to say. Every morning Margery[40] [*sic*] and I retire to our bedrooms & read German either by ourselves or together In the afternoon we usually make some kind of expedition together & get tea out. In the evening we come in to dinner & afterwards sit around in the dining room table with the family playing patience or some-

[40] Marjorie. Adrian was casual about spelling the name correctly.

> thing & trying to talk German. It is dreadfully dull. The people, too, are so stupid. Now that they have got tired of saying how slow & inartistic the English are the only subject, practically, left to them is food.
>
> I hope that you will find some more amusing place for your honeymoon. I had an amazingly characteristic letter from Saxon about the wedding. He gave me a list of all the people who had been at Gordon Square, the order of their arrival at the house and of their departure. Otherwise he had not a single comment to make. I got a better account from Duncan, though, who appears to have been by far the smartest man present with the possible exception of George. It must have been an odd scene, I wish I could have been there. I wonder where you are now. I think you had better come here, won't the Ring tempt you? It can't go on raining much longer I don't think and it wouldn't then be so bad if there were more people one could talk to. However I suppose you will be selfish and go somewhere else.

His feeling for Virginia seems to have become more open and affectionate since the days in Fitzroy Square. In January, 1914, he marked her birthday, January 25.

> My dear Goat
> Many happy returns of the day. You will get an odd parcel which is meant for a birthday present. I couldn't think at all of anything you would like to have but as I walked along the street, I saw them in a shop window and I thought there was just a chance that they might come in useful. They are a pair of slippers and they look warm and in this cold weather I thought they might be some help in keeping off the blains. If they are the wrong size they can be changed. The man told me that the easiest way to put them on was to press the heel part inwards level with the inside of the sole then to slip your foot in over it and afterwards to pull it out again.

Soon after the outbreak of war on August 4, 1914, Adrian wrote to Duncan:

> This war is a perfect nightmare and no-one can talk of anything else. . . . Whether to volunteer or not I cannot quite

make up my mind. You see the French are doing jolly badly and I'm afraid we have got to face the fact that they are very likely to be beaten before the Russians can do much harm in Germany Of course as soon as the Russians get near Berlin the Germans will have to detach part of their army and it is then that the French chance will come again if they can only hold out long enough. Then they will want all the troops we can give them . . . If I am killed, which would be more likely than otherwise, there would be less of an upset in other people's lives than if I were married.

He wrote again:

Karin seems to think that one ought to volunteer and even says she is very depressed wondering whether I am going to do so or fail. However her reasoning is not very sound, it seems to be based on patriotism which is so silly. 'He is not very calm about it either. I don't know what this National reserve is that your father wants you to join . . . I will find out about it. If we are both going to the wars it might be as well for us to go together.'

In the end they both became conscientious objectors as did most of their friends. Before they were all dispersed there was a gathering at a camp organized by Brynhild Olivier at the Lizard. Adrian writes to Duncan:

Bad old Quad
I was wired to by the camp the other day saying that they were breaking up on Wed. 26th so I hopped into the night train on Friday evening & arrived at Helston at 7 o'clock on Saturday. I found there a small pony trap – what they call a 'jingle' – and after about two hours drive arrived here. The other people are Bryn and her baby & Daphne & Maynard & a small boy of 12 called Fergus Maclearey. Everybody else has gone off for one reason or another. Noel to nurse the wounded in a London hospital & Margery[41] to look after the Germans in London! It seems very far from all the war here

[41] Margery Olivier may have been occupied with the German civilians marooned in England. A number, many of them musicians, were interned in considerable discomfort and cold at the Alexandra Palace in North London where they were visited by their English counterparts for whom and with whom they gave concerts. I remember being taken there by my mother.

> and the only news we get is pretty precarious. Falmouth Harbour however which is only a few miles away is crammed full with German shipping which has been captured & we are always seeing the cruisers which are knocking about at the entrance to the Channel on the look out for more . . . Last night we sat round the camp fire & talked about love and kissing & I told them the story of Margery Olivier and Margery Rosenbaum with great success. These young ladies however seem to have a queer prejudice against kissing though intellectually they quite approve of it – it is quite instructive.

The significance of kissing at the time can hardly be exaggerated. A man in conventional middle-class circles who kissed a girl might be forced by her irate father to marry her. In a review of Jonathan Gathorne Hardy's biography of Gerald Brenan the reviewer makes the point that in Edwardian England 'making love' could mean anything from flirting to sexual intercourse.[42] And there were degrees of kissing: on the mouth would be unacceptably 'fast'. (A member of the Bloomsbury Group with a reputation for his conquests told a friend that glimpsing a pretty girl at the other end of the corridor in a train he had had an erection. This he referred to as having 'had her'!)

Adrian took a delight in kissing and placed an emphasis on it that puzzled Karin when, towards the end of 1914, he began to be interested in her, making a second attempt at a serious relationship with a woman. Karin was very different from Noel. The story of her courtship and marriage is told in her diary, written between 1913 and 1915.

[42] *London Review of Books*, August 20, 1992.

12

KARIN COSTELLOE

Karin Costelloe was born in 1889, descended on her mother's side from a Philadelphia Quaker family.

Her mother, Mary Whitall Smith, was the daughter of the formidable Hannah Whitall Smith, who held views about the subjection of women that are relevant today. When Mary announced her engagement to Frank Costelloe, an Irish barrister who had been staying with the Smiths while attending meetings of the American Association of Science in Philadelphia, Hannah's objection was not so much to Frank himself, though his Catholicism dismayed her, as to husbands in general. Men, she believed, were 'very jealous of their rights and are unwilling to allow any freedom of action or development to their wives . . . I believe in a perfect equality between husband and wife as between man and woman . . . I am convinced that most of the misery in married life arises from the fact that, unconsciously perhaps, the soul of the woman is chafing against the tyranny of sex.'[43]

But Mary stood firm. In 1885 Hannah, now thoroughly alarmed, took the whole family to England, her husband Robert, Mary and her sister Alys, cousin Madge Whitall, and Logan who was to spend the winter in Berlin studying German. When Hannah saw that the engagement was a *fait accompli* she consented to the marriage which took place in September 1885 at Balliol with due ceremony and presided over by the illustrious Benjamin Jowett.

Mary and Frank bought a house in Pimlico, 40 Grosvenor Road, lavishly furnished by Mary's parents. Her first pregnancy ended in a miscarriage; but a daughter, Rachel, was born in June 1887. Mary did not want another child, but Catholic methods of birth control, principally abstinence, failed and an unwanted child, Catherine Elizabeth (Karin) was born in March 1889.

[43] Barbara Halpern Strachey, *Remarkable Relations.*

During the summer of 1890 Bernard Berenson came to London and was invited by the Costelloes to Friday's Hill Cottage, their house in Surrey, for the Bank Holiday. Mary, looking back much later, noted in her diary, 'Fascinated I listened to his talk about Provençal poetry, about the Greek Anthology . . . I felt like a dry sponge that was put in water. Instinctively I realised these were the real values for me, however wicked and self-indulgent they might be.'[44] At first Frank found him excellent company but as Mary's love for Berenson became obvious he demurred at their constant association; and Mary's determination to join Bernard in Italy was more than he could tolerate. Anxious to avoid a scandal he acquiesced in her spending the winter in Florence, even to her taking the children with her. She brought them home in May. But when she returned to Italy alone, the breach between them widened. The ensuing turmoil centred round the children. Frank wanted custody and for them to be brought up in the Catholic Church. When discussing the children Karin was mentioned only to suggest that if she could keep Ray he could keep Karin.

In 1895, Frank had contracted cancer of the ear. Realising that he might die he made a will excluding Mary and everyone in her family from guardianship of the children and disinheriting them if his wishes were not complied with (he had left them £200 each). A friendly priest told Hannah of this and she had them made Wards in Chancery. When Frank died in September 1895, Hannah had to go to Law to get custody of the children and to guarantee them enough securities to ensure that they each got an annual income of £200.

For the children life with Hannah was happier and more stable. She removed them from a second-rate convent school to a good day-school, Kensington High School for Girls. From the beginning Mary had doted on Ray, virtually ignoring Karin, perhaps because she had been unwanted; or because of her likeness to her father; and there was Ray's equable nature compared with Karin's which was excitable and unpredictable. Moreover, Karin was beginning to suffer from agonising ear-ache – she had to undergo five operations before she was eighteen – it is not surprising that she grew up 'hasty, tactless, emotional and rowdy'.

In 1907, Karin followed Ray to Newnham, which Ray enjoyed. But Karin was miserable, isolated by her deafness. Mary thought the Cambridge climate was bad for her; also, the best lip-reading

[44] Ibid.

teachers were in America. In the autumn of 1908 she and Bernard left for America on another client-finding tour, taking both girls and Ray's friend, Elly Strachey, who were to spend a year at Bryn Mawr. Karin thoroughly enjoyed her time there, responding to the warmth and friendliness of her numerous relations. She flung herself into parties and dances and discovered the satisfaction of demanding work. Carey Thomas, Dean of Studies, encouraged her to read philosophy and psychology, both taught at Bryn Mawr. 'It is positively a life-work', Karin wrote home, 'and when you go into it with close attention a lot of it is very unsatisfactory and vague. Of course psychology is only at its initial stage and they can only talk vaguely about it.'

Karin returned to Newnham to take her tripos, changing her subject to Moral Sciences. Bertrand Russell, her uncle by his marriage to Alys Pearsall Smith, a lecturer at Trinity College, hearing her spoken of very highly by her tutors, decided to coach her himself. And in 1910 she gained first-class honours. He wrote to her, 'I am overjoyed to hear you have got a First. Considering how little time you have had for working at the subject, it is a remarkable feat . . . You have a real aptitude for philosophy, and I expect that Part II will suit you even better than Part I.'

On June 24, 1911, he wrote again congratulating her on her starred First in Part II. He approved of her plan to continue post-graduate work. She must learn to work independently 'at a theme that interests you. You must learn German and read the books on it. Write a treatise of, say, 50,000 words on your subject before showing it to anyone. That is what fellowship candidates do and it seems to me the right plan. When it is done I shall be glad to read it and criticise it; but you won't acquire originality unless you work without help for a bit.'

Thus inspired Karin began her dissertation on Henri Bergson's philosophy, which was eventually to become her book, *The Misuse of Mind*, published in 1922. On February 5, 1913, she began her diary.

'Some theorists', she wrote, 'love logical consistency rather than truth – it's a Cambridge tendency and I don't share it.' A group photograph of the Moral Sciences Club in 1913 shows her on the right at the end of the front row, with her fine dark head of hair and her legs demurely crossed under her long skirt. (The Whitall women had legs like Greek columns.) 'Uncle Bertie' sits in the centre of the same row; G. E. Moore is third from the right at the end of the third row. 'I like her,' Bertrand Russell wrote to a friend. 'She's a nice girl if only she were not so graceless.'

Karin was handsome, with glossy, abundant hair and true Irish blue eyes, and an alert response to conversation which interested her. But her clumsiness in childhood had persisted, and her rather heavy body was at odds with her agile brain. She loved clothes, but her taste was uncoordinated and her choice of colour flamboyant. As her family inheritance, manic depression, increased, the contrast between her low spirits and fits of weeping and her boisterous gaiety became more marked.

Karin's work was enlivened by her introduction to the Bloomsbury set through her sister Ray, who had married Oliver Strachey in 1911. In 1913, Lytton Strachey had written to Henry Lamb about a Bloomsbury fancy dress party given by Oliver on June 23: 'Karin was the leading figure, in white flannel cricketing trousers and shirt. . . . The gambols were extraordinary and in the middle of them Gerald [Shove] appeared, drunk, in evening dress and a top-hat. He and Karin sang a Vesta Tilley song together and carried on a great deal. I was considerably in love with them both.'

Even before Karin completed her thesis, there is evidence of the interest in abnormal psychology which was to absorb her in later years. For instance, on February 22, 1914, she wrote to Duncan, asking him to send books of the kind recommended by Clive Bell. One title was *Coups de Fouet* (Whip Lashes) and 'anything interesting' about *Fassades* (Spanking). Her nascent interests included homosexuality, or 'Topic No. 2' as she called it.

Later that year she herself, with her friend Hope Mirrlees,[45] visited Paris where she showed her work to Henri Bergson. He approved of her critique and they became friends. She invited Duncan Grant to tea at L'Hotel d'Elysée to meet Gertrude Stein, Monsieur Vildrac[46] (a well-known poet) and Madame Bergson.

Karin finished her thesis in May; it was accepted and she won her fellowship at Newnham. She was free to pursue her interest in 'Topic No. 2'. Her flat in Great Ormond Street was a short walk from 38 Brunswick Square and the communal ménage, now augmented by Gerald Shove, who had taken the rooms vacated by Leonard Woolf. Duncan Grant she knew reasonably well; Maynard Keynes she had first met at I Tatti in 1907 when her mother, anxious

45 A writer and poet. The Hogarth Press published a volume of her poetry. Virginia Woolf thought her pretentious and affected but she was a good friend to Karin. 'She believes in me.'

46 Charles Vildrac, French dramatist, poet and art critic (1882–1971).

to find suitable husbands for the girls, had applied to Aunt Lou (Alys Russell). She had dispatched Geoffrey Scott, a young man of no particular bent, though he wrote poetry, and Maynard Keynes, then a young man at King's. Karin disliked Geoffrey Scott, though he fell in love with her, but she liked Maynard, and he took to her. Karin had never fallen in love with anyone, though she longed for a romantic involvement.

What remains of her diary is in poor condition, passages indecipherable or completely erased. Towards the end of the summer of 1914 she wrote:

> This year has been the most lovely time for me. I finished off my thesis in a frenzy at the beginning of May and since then I have been taken up and stalked by Topic No. 2 with silent tread, till now I can distinctly hear the sounds of thunderous feet. (I am installed in the heart of the fraternity.) They are all such dears and are fond of me and are pleased to have me around so that I love it and am in a warm douche of pleasure and wish them well with my whole heart. Ray's party began the season. That was nicest at the time when, flushed with brandy and soda I allowed myself to put my arm round Duncan's neck and *tutoi*[47] him. They are right in saying that Duncan, *Le Ciel* as Hope and I called him in Paris, is like a flower. It doesn't matter what he does or says (fortunately for he puts this continually to the test) he is incorruptibly pure. I have a feeling about him which isn't the least being in love, but makes me feel fully contented when he is there and rather sad when he is absent. It's not much use getting him to care about me they say he is hopelessly Topic No. 2. All the same I think he is fond of me in his remote childish way . . . Yesterday I made him have supper with me in the Park and we got on rather well. . . . I had asked him in order to have him to myself. . . . He, however, made me come round right after to Gordon Square where all the others were sitting around. . . . He partly wanted to please Adrian who is a little bit in love with me. It was never anything much with him until my party. That was an amazing affair. It was given to celebrate my getting my fellowship and I had invited Maynard, Duncan, Gerald, Vanessa, Clive and Adrian. . . . We were all very gay. I could not go near Maynard . . . without having my leg caressed. I made no

[47] Tutoyer. Use of the second person singular indicates a degree of familiarity.

> secret of being a keen student of Topic No. 2 of which I took all this to be the signs. Besides I am fond of Maynard, funny, gentle-eyed satyr. . . . The demonstrations got more pronounced as the port circulated freely. Finally I went into the kitchen to fill a jug of water and to my amazement was kissed. I laughed and called him silly and we tottered back on the best of understandings. Their methods are more civilised than those of Topic No. 1. Their talk is so light and there is very charming comradeship. . . . He let me alone for a while but when I fell exhausted on a sofa after dancing he put his arm round me. He is a satyr. I had to keep his hands carefully on neutral ground. . . . But he was gentle and easily controlled. . . . Then he pulled me on to his knees. . . . Adrian said he would if I liked . . . I said I was quite ready but he was comically shy. We went into the other room and Maynard began kissing my hand passionately . . . Maynard was getting more and more excited. He told me he was drunk. . . . He spoke to me . . . as to my possible Topic No. 2 subject. He and Adrian both wanted to kiss me good-night a great many times before Oliver[48] finally got them away.
>
> That really started Adrian off a little. He would very much like me to do it again, but I can't make a practice of that sort of thing.

On another occasion, she had returned from a party with Duncan to Brunswick Square, where they found Adrian, Gerald Shove and Maynard.

> Adrian spent the evening urging me to kiss people as a sort of 8th work of mercy because he said they would enjoy it so. We laughed a lot and he walked home with me in the dawn. It was very beautiful. I wonder whether I tease too much; my behaviour is rather monstrous but somehow I believe it's all right. It's all so lighthearted and somehow I don't think he will fall badly in love. If he doesn't it's surely great fun for him too. I think he takes his risks gladly so it is not my affair to act as governess to either of us.

The previous night when they had come in from Gordon Square Garden she walked round to Brunswick Square with

[48] Oliver Strachey had married Ray Costelloe.

Duncan and Saxon. Karin agreed to come in for just one more drink. Presumably in Adrian's bedroom, 'he flung himself upon me to try and put me in. We had a glorious tangle . . . and I nearly lost a tooth. This put us in the best spirits.'

The beginning of the war, on August 4, 1914, seems to have had little influence on their behaviour or their decisions. It is hard to find a time when they turned from being play-fellows to serious consideration about their relationship. In 1914 Adrian was thirty-one, Karin twenty-five. We have no means of knowing what Adrian thought at the time. But from her diary, which seeks to recall honestly her own confused and fluctuating deliberations, enough may be gathered to surmise his extreme confusion and uncertainty, his attempted withdrawals and his ultimate exhaustion and compliance. At no time could they be considered 'lovers'; yet their behaviour led friends and family to suppose they might be, and to watch with increasing dismay, since no one thought Karin was 'the right person' for Adrian.

Adrian and Karin spent a week together at Asheham towards the end of August. They were hardly ever apart 'except the very few hours that were left for sleep'. After the others had gone to bed they sat on in the study or went on long walks in the dawn, 'sometimes talking about ourselves or each other, sometimes just kissing'. Once, returning from a walk to Newhaven, she 'gave him my own first tentative kiss, whereupon Adrian discovered kissing on the lips . . . I felt steadily more and more uneasy.' He was, she felt, 'experimenting in the dark with something that would end by hurting him'.

The evening before they left Asheham they 'sat soberly apart, but in this novel position they could find nothing to say. Adrian was in a most engaging "half-witted" mood which appealed very much to my affection.'

As they left next day 'a fresh trouble came in the shape of Duncan's grief. Adrian had tears in his eyes as we got into the cab and I felt miserable because I felt sure I was going to bring unhappiness to them both.'

Back in Brunswick Square her deliberations continued; it was an increasingly wretched, sleepless time for them both. 'I felt rather dazed all the time and curiously dead.' She told him she respected and admired him more than anyone she had met, but did not love him. Would he take her on these terms, hoping that love would come? 'He said he hardly knew but did not think I had better take on so much of a risk.' She chewed over the idea and 'it began to seem to me a good thing to marry Adrian if he would have me without my being in love, but I was uneasy still. It would be so wretched never to be in love happily.'

If their sleeplessness and tension made Adrian less communicative, it had the opposite effect on Karin, who weighed up the pros and cons as they sat, night after night, on Adrian's sofa. But her idea of a loveless marriage based on mutual respect and esteem seems to have given her some sort of impetus, for the following day they went down to Ford Place in Sussex, a house belonging to Logan and Alys where Mary Berenson stayed on her visits to England.

The carriage was empty, and she was 'very much kissed' all the way. 'Mother came to meet us in a great white hat and dress. She little thought she was meeting her future son-in-law, nor did I.' After the others had gone to bed, her deliberations continued, in spite of the usual kissing. Finally she 'came out with "Adrian I will marry you if you want me to." He asked me if I meant it . . . I answered that I wasn't in love with him and burst into tears . . . I think I wanted him to put his arms round me and simply tell me he wanted me to marry him. But . . . he behaved like an angel and would not let me escape the responsibility of deciding for myself . . . . When I urged him at last he said he advised me to marry him. I had worn him out completely so that he was quite pale and too dazed to mind about anything.'

Her mother persuaded her not to have a long engagement since she had to take up her fellowship and wouldn't be able to work till all was settled. They were married in the Register Office in the St George's Hanover Square District, on October 31, 1914. The witnesses were Mary Berenson and Duncan Grant. They immediately left for Cornwall.

Honeymoons are all too often an unhappy way to begin married life, specially when women were supposed to be virgins, as Karin was. Adrian took her to St Ives, so full of memories for him of idealised family life. It rained a good deal; and Karin wept continuously. Adrian offered to divorce her when they returned to wartime Cambridge where she took up her fellowship. But Karin, in spite of her manic-depressive tendency and her perpetual earache, was stout-hearted and determined to make something of their marriage, as was Adrian. Work, as always, was her antidote. They rented a flat in Hoop Lane, once a hotel, now converted with shops below, near Emmanuel College. They led a reasonably social life, since Karin was fêted by her Cambridge friends and colleagues, among whom she was always at her best, and Adrian had friends and family connections there. No more is recorded about his work for Vinogradoff[49] which, presumably, had been cut short by the war, and the decimation of most of his students on the Western Front.

[49] Vinogradoff, a radical, returned to Russia in 1917, enthusiastically welcoming the Revolution. Eventually, disillusioned, he returned to Oxford.

13

CONSCIENTIOUS OBJECTOR

Karin took up her diary again on January 15, 1915: 'Adrian and I have been married a year last October and I am expecting my first baby in a month. So that is how it all turned out and I am so glad.'

This sets the tone of their affectionate domesticity. They were seen walking about Cambridge hand in hand. Pernel Strachey, a don at Newnham, remarked that 'the lofty Adrian and the short, stolid Karin looked like a tall giraffe looking down and a young bird poking up.' Karin, as she noted in her diary, was still subject to fits of weeping. How much these bouts of despair were due to the manic-depressive tendency she had inherited and how much to the uncertainties of her relationship with Adrian is impossible to guess.

Their material comfort would have been greater but for Karin's total ignorance of domestic matters. Virginia Woolf commented in her diary, 'I had a request from Adrian for silver, glass and kitchen things. He wrote by a candle light stuck in a saucer.' After Alys Russell had paid them a visit she described the chaos, slops unemptied, beds unmade, clothes and books all over the place. But carpets and furniture were bought, curtains ordered from the Omega Workshop, servants interviewed.

Adrian wrote occasional articles for the Selden Society, and later one on a pamphlet of Leslie Stephen's was accepted by the *Cambridge Magazine* and published in November 1917. But he had never earned a regular income. Mary and Bernhard Berenson, the chief source of their income, were so outraged by their taking an 'unpatriotic' stand on conscientious objection that they threatened to cut off all financial support. Mary had never given her daughters a regular allowance but she made them generous, even lavish, gifts and paid for any extra expenses such as the cost of Karin's ear operations; and she could be depended upon to dispense dollops of cash fairly regularly. Adrian had been left £200 by his aunt, Emilia Stephen, and other sources are alluded to from time to time by Adrian who took charge of the family affairs. Jack Hills made them all an allowance and on his death they could each expect a share in Stella's considerable Duckworth fortune.

Karin had £200 a year settled on her by her grandmother and the grant for her Newnham Fellowship was £160 per annum. But the bulk of their income came from the Berensons, a dependence which with their radical beliefs they deplored but accepted, not always with good grace. However, the threat of losing it did not materialise and they continued to live a reasonably comfortable life. They entertained occasionally and made the most of Cambridge wartime society in spite of its being depressing. While Karin worked on her book on Bergson's philosophy Adrian was for a time uncertain what to do. From Hoop Chambers late in 1914 he wrote to Duncan, who was thinking of joining an ambulance unit, that he too might consider joining a Quaker ambulance unit. He and Karin had agreed that he, Adrian, ought to do something about 'the crisis . . . This isn't patriotism but simply that things seem to be in such an awful mess, and there isn't a great deal to do in my own job. I don't suppose the Selden Society will be publishing for a bit.'

In his next letter he had found a new, promising occupation working for the Union of Democratic Control. The UDC was founded in September 1914 by those who opposed entry into the war to ensure that the secret diplomatic errors, which were in their view the cause of the war, should not be repeated. Among other influential members of the UDC were Ramsay MacDonald and Bertrand Russell. The latter was fined for a pamphlet which allegedly discouraged recruiting and was deprived of his Fellowship – restored in 1944. The secretary, C. D. Morel, a journalist and writer, was imprisoned for sending printed matter to a neutral country.

Adrian's work for the UDC encouraged his radical beliefs. When he found a cause that engaged his sympathies he was by no means the passive, indolent individual he is often represented as being. From Hoop Chambers, in a letter to Duncan Grant postmarked 27 April, 1915, he wrote: 'My work at the UDC goes on & I have collected 20 people now to write letters to the papers. Hardly a day goes by now without a letter appearing over my name in some paper in London or the country. It is rather comic isn't it? Sometimes I get several headlines calling me a Traitor & all sorts of names.'

Adrian was also on the committee of the National Council for Civil Liberties (formerly the National Council against Conscription). He wrote to Leonard Woolf on August 10, 1915, that the NCCL might have a vacancy for secretary as the present secretary, Langdon Davies, had been conscripted. (Virginia Woolf wrote in her diary, 'Karin wants to remove him from the UDC. The work is too elementary.' Karin failed. But it is an indication of the arbitrary control she had begun to exert over Adrian which was one reason for her unpopularity among his friends.)

An entry in the college Annual Register (1915) records that Karin had resigned her Fellowship 'as she was obliged for reasons unconnected with her work to leave Cambridge and live in London. She had not been able to begin the work she had hoped to undertake concerning abnormal psychology as throwing light on memory and personality. She has drafted the scheme for a book on Bergson's philosophy which she hopes to publish later, and has written the introductory chapter. She has also read a paper to the Aristotelian Society on Complexity and Synthesis and Comparisons of the Data and Philosophical Method of Mr Russell and Monsieur Bergson.'

In May 1915 she and Adrian took a short holiday in Dorset. They wanted to live in London, but must avoid staying with 'Auntie Lou she does rub it in so'. They might go to a Bloomsbury hotel. There is something wraithlike about these two wandering in the mist and rain, uncertain of their future. Though conscription was not imposed until 1916 their friends were prepared for it. Desmond MacCarthy was said to be driving an ambulance in France. Later he joined the Naval Reserve, working in the Intelligence Department at the Admiralty. Oliver Strachey, aged forty, was at the Foreign Office in the code and deciphering department. (He and Ray supported the war.) Leonard Woolf would get exemption on health grounds, as would Lytton Strachey. Maynard Keynes was with Saxon Sydney-Turner at the Treasury on work of national importance. Duncan Grant and David Garnett became self-employed agricultural labourers cared for by Vanessa Bell, first at Wissett Lodge in Suffolk. When Vanessa took Charleston farmhouse in Firle, West Sussex, Duncan and David Garnett found employment near by. Clive was given farmwork at Garsington. His anti-war pamphlet, *Peace at Once*, published in the spring of 1915, was destroyed by the Lord Mayor of London, outraging his father who threatened to cut him off from the family.

But Adrian had still not decided what to do. He wrote to Duncan that Karin had urged that he, Adrian, should do 'something to help the War effort, not fight but something useful'. He might drive an ambulance. By the time he was called up a year later he had decided to work on the land. With his law training he was able to attend tribunals and act for his friends who were conscientious objectors. He was least successful when representing Duncan and David Garnett at their tribunal in Wissett. They failed to get exemption from military service. Naturally, Keynes was delighted. 'Adrian had presented their case very badly, as though he was addressing a judge in Chancery.' In mid-July their case was heard in Ipswich. This time Maynard was in command. Impressive, with Treasury aplomb, he swept in, demanding that 'their case should be heard promptly – he had left urgent business of the utmost national importance'.[50] The two got their exemption.

For a short time Adrian and Karin lodged with friends at Sandwell, near Radlett, Hertfordshire. But late in May they rented part of 31 Bedford Square. Air-raids had begun in 1914, when the first Zeppelin crossed over the British coast on December 23, 1914, gliding through the clouds like a silver pencil; the apparition was awe-inspiring. When it was discovered that the lighter-than-air ships were vulnerable, being slow and filled with hydrogen so that they were shot down in flames by the Royal Flying Corps, they were followed by aeroplane attacks.

No one had ever before been bombarded from the air, and there was a certain amount of panic. One Zeppelin fell near Potters Bar; and it was said that a 'Hun', falling through the flames, was 'so fat he dented the ground', a legend that provoked hilarity and jubilation. War hysteria and a hate campaign were whipped up by press and government to counteract the truth, the full horror of trench warfare in a conflict ill-prepared and callously ill-led by 'the Generals' backed by the government, a war which gathered its own appallingly unstoppable momentum. Surprisingly, when Adrian wrote to Vanessa from 31 Bedford Square on May 20, 1915, he did not mention Zeppelins.

> We had our first air raid last night. The warning went off about 11 o'clock and we did not get the all clear till about half-past one. I don't think many bombs were dropped very close to us but the guns made an awful row and you could hear the engines of the aeroplanes apparently quite near by.

[50] *Maynard Keynes* by Robert Skidelsky

> They seemed to come in about four detachments and between each there was a short lull when you thought it was all over but in about 10 minutes it all broke out again. At last we did get the 'All Clear' but before they had finished sounding it the maroons started exploding again & the sirens hooting for a second warning. Mercifully they did not come again this time. It did not seem really alarming but it is not very pleasant to have the banging going on. I am more frightened that it may affect Karin in her present condition [she was pregnant] than of anything else. However she keeps amazingly cool.

Karin worked with Adrian at the National Council Against Conscription. As 'conchies' they got rough treatment from bystanders. 'Coming out from the office with Bob Trevelyan and Gerald Shove a "rough" suddenly turned and hit Bob full on the mouth. A woman scooped up some mud and threw it at my face. Others set on me from behind. Some struck at Adrian till he was quite giddy. Another shouted at Gerald, "bloody German!" and knocked him out. Police stood by without intervening. Uncle Bertie is anxious to bear testimony and get jailed, but they don't seem to want him.'

In spite of her rough handling Karin's pregnancy was not impaired, and on January 23, 1916, probably at Sandwell, their daughter Ann was born. 'She has a nurse, Elsie, who, though she is deaf, is reliable, and a splendid pram,' Karin wrote to her mother. As there was no room for the pram at 31 Bedford Square, Lady Ottoline Morrell agreed to keep it in her hall until they had a permanent home.

They sublet their flat in Bedford Square, and were hopeful of finding a house in Hampstead. On July 27, they moved into 29 Tanza Road, a large, airy house with a view over Parliament Hill Fields.

Later that month Adrian appeared before his local tribunal. He was given twenty-one days to find work on the land. Karin writes to her mother with a mixture of contempt and irritation: 'He would like doing it and I think it would be very good for his health and it would of course solve the whole question of what is to become of him.'

In August Adrian found work at Stud Farm, Prestonbury, near Cheltenham. There were two farms, one run by a Mrs Gardiner. At first they were amalgamated, later run separately. From there on September 24 he wrote to Duncan: 'I only wish we could make a place for you here.' He was kept busy digging in the fields; much of his time was spent milking. 'I am not a great hand at milking yet, but I'm getting better.'

They moved into a farmhouse which they set about furnishing to accommodate themselves and their workers, a household that was to include Gerald Shove, the economist, and his wife, Fredegond, a poet. 'I think that will be rather fun.'

The Shoves did not think it was fun. They were appalled at the discomfort, the dirt, the chaotic squalor of the farmhouse. Fredegond Shove wrote to Vanessa: 'It was lovely of you to write. Adrian told Gerald he very nearly steamed open the letter. I am glad he didn't for he might have guessed how much I hate [three words illegible]. Poor old Karin has been having a bad time with her ears – she is very brave. Adrian looks too beautiful to be true in his pale, fawn velvet and is, I think, almost the best person in the world.'

Karin, meanwhile, had already taken a more elaborate view of their venture. They were considering turning the two farms into a limited company with Mrs Gardiner, plans which were interrupted by a bitter quarrel with B.B. Upset by their pacifism, he threatened to withold their 'wedding present' of £500. (Somewhat delayed.) But Mary Berenson arranged matters, or paid the money herself. Karin, thanking her, wrote that it was a relief for they had already promised the £500 as part of the loan capital.

Karin was forever on the move; Adrian became less buoyant. Matters did not go smoothly on the farm. They and Mrs Gardiner parted company. A new manager was brought in and wanted the house they had just moved into. To add to the gloom, Jasper, their dog, was run over. There were still no customers for babies' pure milk, though Mrs Gardiner offered to sell it through 'a big farmers' union'.

On October 26, 1916, Adrian wrote to Vanessa from Prestonbury:

> We have had such a business getting this farm going & so on that we could not very well embark on taking another house just now especially as it seemed quite possible that Karin's income might be very much cut down owing to our quarrel with B.B. The running of this farm is going to be a bigger job

even than we expected. There are troubles about wages for the men who have some of them got families to support & are accustomed to a standard of living they can no longer afford now. Then there are difficulties about servants as it has got about that we are C.O.s it is rather hard to find people to do for the men. I myself do not have a great deal of time to deal with outside troubles as I begin work about 6 and don't get off until about 6 in the evening with about 2 hrs for meals.

However, it isn't all quite as black as it sounds. I don't really mind the work at all, in fact I rather enjoy dealing with the animals. I am gradually becoming quite a competent milker & can milk easily 7 or 8 cows every morning and afternoon. I shall soon be competent to do more but that is all I have time to do at the pace I can go at present. I expect you hve heard terrible tales of our life from Gerald because as far as I can gather he has been going about saying all sorts of things about us. The truth is, I think, that he found the work a great deal harder for him than he expected and he got thoroughly uninterested & eventually found that his conscience didn't allow him to stay on. I wasn't very sorry as he never really got through his share which made things harder for the rest of us, though it was pleasant to have some one civilised to talk to sometimes.

By December they were considering possible plans to move. Adrian wrote to Vanessa on December 10 that he would like to go to work for Philip Morrell at Garsington if his tribunal would allow him. Philip is 'very anxious to get some one to milk his cows'. Also, 'when we thought there would be no difficulty in our way we arranged to take a house so that if we don't go we shall have to get rid of it.' They had had to give up their house to the new manager, and he had to get up at six o'clock and bicycle to work – a hardship on these frosty mornings.

The tribunal did not allow him to get to Garsington. But on January 17, 1917 he wrote from Ray Strachey's house that he had just rung up the tribunal and been granted permission to work for the Phillimores[51] so, instead of returning to Cheltenham they went back to Radlett to inspect yet another new house.

[51] Robert Charles Phillimore (1871-1919) of Kendall Hall, near Aldenham (in the Radlett area) was a barrister and Lord of the Manor. His was one of the two principal landowning families in that part. 'Lion' Phillimore was a friend of Alys and Bertrand Russell. ('Lion' was her nickname.)

Once settled at Radlett, they addressed the serious question of taking over Henry, a dog, from Duncan at Charleston. Now they were only thirty-five minutes by train from London, they could come quite often. They enjoyed bridge with Ka and a friend; and Karin read a paper at Cambridge to the Aristotelian Society on Bergson's philosophy. They had dinner with 'Goldie'.[52] Bertrand Russell 'flew at Karin like a terrier. He passionately hated all she said. But Karin stood firm.' On one of their bridge evenings Adrian fell back in his chair in a dead faint.

Towards the end of 1917 he became seriously ill. Dr Buzzard, an eminent specialist, diagnosed severe exhaustion from physical labour, and imminent heart failure. Total breakdown could only be avoided by at least six months' rest. Surely, Karin hoped, a diagnosis from so distinguished a medical man would influence the tribunal. After some demur he was allowed to take up less demanding work, as secretary on the Phillimore estate. Adrian wrote again to Vanessa: 'A very pleasant change after digging. I have to do very little except keep farm books, go to the bank and pay wages and so on, and I am almost done by lunch time . . . Ann is getting such a size that though she is only a year and ten months she can hardly wear clothes that are supposed to be for a child of three and a half.'

Adrian was fond of his nephews Julian and Quentin. He loved fun, acting a part, teasing – all of which appealed to them. Quentin recalled an incident when he and his brother were playing in the top flat at 50 Gordon Square, misbehaving with an airgun, 'and considerable irresponsibility'. Suddenly they were arrested by a deep voice behind them: 'I am taking you to the police station!' Adrian, very tall, very serious, very alarming.

Another aspect of his character appealed to his nephews: he was a gambler, not just at poker, but when driving a car, or sailing. He took hair-raising though never quite death-dealing risks. Once, when Adrian was taking Quentin and his mother for a drive, they had just topped the brow of a hill and began to descend when the engine failed. 'Put your foot on that brake pedal and keep it there,' he told Vanessa, as he got out to investigate. 'What will happen if I take it off?' she called out as he crawled under the engine. 'I shall be killed.' (Why hadn't he secured the handbrake? Perhaps he had, and enjoyed the sensation he hoped to cause?)

52 Goldsworthy Lowes Dickinson was a Fellow of King's College and an Apostle. He was a longstanding proponent of international understanding and coined the name 'League of Nations'.

They returned to Tanza Road in February, 1918. Adrian, still unwell, was no longer obliged to do war work. But Karin was now feeling the strain of the past five years. 'I feel utterly exhausted with making and unmaking plans.' Her ears were bad, she was pregnant, the veins in her legs were troublesome. Unwelcome though they probably were, the whole family descended on Leonard and Virginia at Asheham. Rooms were found for Adrian and Karin near by. But Ann, aged two, and her nurse Daisy, had to live in the house; they all had their meals there. Matters may have been eased by Daisy being Lottie's sister, part of the network that sustained Stephens, Bells and Woolfs. But it says much for Leonard's tolerance for Virginia's sake.

The two brothers-in-law had never got on well except on political and social questions such as the UDC, the Labour Party and the League of Nations. One of Leonard's closest friends had been Thoby, in that charmed circle which excluded others. 'The wrong man died.' This haunting conviction may have contributed to Adrian's coolness. But what really worsened their relations was Leonard's dislike of Karin. He could hardly bear her in the house.

Out walking with Virginia, Adrian spoke of Karin, her bouts of depression, her deafness. He was proud of her vitality, so wanting in himself.

Some three months before her confinement Karin had an abdominal operation. But she recovered in time for Judith's birth on November 7, 1918. Adrian wrote to Vanessa and Duncan, 'Another girl. A disappointment of course. Karin so much wants a boy we think of trying again.' He wrote in some detail about the birth. He was with her all the time. She had twilight sleep: 'the pains owing to the operation became fearfully intense very early on. . . . You could see quite clearly that she would not have stood them for very much longer. She was having the most ghastly pains every few minutes and they injected the stuff and she went to sleep quite quietly for some hours. By the way, the doctor gave us a bottle of chloroform to use in case of desperate hurry.'

On January 17, 1919, three months after Judith's birth, he wrote to Vanessa commiserating her over the difficulty of getting domestic staff. 'We are gradually getting into smoother waters here.' Karin had had an operation on her ear with the hope of improving her hearing. 'I got Karin away from the nursing home which was a perfect Hell of a place. Every conceivable thing went wrong. . . . Now she is back here and feeling much more comfortable. It is too early to say whether the operation has been a success but the surgeon is very pleased with it and I think it has probably done some good though we don't dare to hope for too much . . . Judith promises to be a very large and healthy child which is something to the good.'

The servant problem was as serious as ever. In almost every letter Adrian commiserates with Vanessa on her lack of adequate help, and regrets searches made without success. He and Karin have their own troubles: Mabel, the children's nurse, wants to rejoin her husband.

The middle classes were perpetually plagued by the dearth of satisfactory servants. The Stephens and the Woolfs swapped them like helots. Vanessa being pregnant, Virginia offered her Lottie and Nelly. Leonard was reluctant to part with them without the assurance that they would return after the birth. (Angelica was born on Christmas Day, 1918.)

From Tanza Road in April, 1919, Karin wrote to her mother that she and Adrian have had a long talk about psychoanalysis with James Strachey and Alix Sargent-Florence, who were to marry the following year. James had recently consulted Ernest Jones about entering the profession. They had also met W. W. Rivers, the anthropologist. Rivers himself never trained as an analyst though his treatment of shell-shocked officers at Craiglockhart in Edinburgh, among them Siegfried Sassoon and Wilfred Owen, owed much to analytical methods at the time. Karin 'settled down to a long talk with Rivers about savages and primitive races. Ethnology is his principal interest.'

(Karin's way of 'settling down to a long talk' with anyone who caught her interest, to the exclusion of everyone else, may have been at least partly due to her deafness, her need to concentrate on one person both to hear and to communicate her own interest. She was always afraid of being left out, of not making and keeping friends.)

In June Karin wrote of their determination to become psychoanalysts. As a necessary preliminary they had to study medicine and had entered their names at University College Hospital. 'We are both absolutely determined to get to the bottom of abnormal psychology and to practise as psychoanalysts. . . . Adrian is reading Morton Prince's *Disassociation of A Personality* . . . What is so jolly is Adrian's passionate enthusiasm about his new work. . . . He is naturally a scientist but got into the wrong boat because of his father's literary tastes, which made him educate Adrian mistakenly.'

In June Virginia wrote to Vanessa: 'I dropped in on Adrian and Karin the other night', (they were still living in Tanza Road) 'to find them scrubbing their saucepans in the kitchen in rather a surly mood; but having done they explained that they are now both to become medical students at University Hospital [*sic*]. They've given up law, philosophy and all the rest of it; they are going into practice together as analysts.'

14

MEDICINE AND PSYCHOANALYSIS

In 1919, when Adrian and Karin began their analysis with James Glover, psychoanalysis was in a transitional state of crisis, of creative upheaval, as Freud's revolutionary theories and discoveries about the workings and structure of the mind continued to pour forth from Berggasse 19, Vienna. His training in the natural sciences and neurology had led him to pursue his own researches into the causes and treatment of neurotic disorders in a scientific spirit. He evolved a technique which enabled him through his work with his patients, confirmed by his own self-analysis, to map out a construct of the workings of the mind. Most significantly he discovered the existence of a subliminal layer of mental activity inaccessible to the conscious mind over which, nevertheless, it has continuous influence. This he called the Unconscious, and it became a basic tenet in the theory and practice of psychoanalysis.

Not surprisingly, considering the emotionally charged nature of their involvement, Freud's followers frequently disagreed, quarrelled or split off to form their own groups. But by 1919 the new 'science' was beginning to coalesce round some of Freud's most able adherents in Berlin, Budapest and Great Britain. In Berlin Karl Abraham, who had attracted a group of brilliant men and women about him, was planning his polyclinic, the first of its kind, with the support of Max Eitingon; it opened in 1920. In Budapest the young Melanie Klein was elected to the Hungarian society after a period of analysis with Ferenczi. She then joined Abraham who encouraged her in her analysis of children.

In Great Britain the prime mover was Dr Ernest Jones who founded the British Psychoanalytical Society in 1919. Faced with an unknown number of individuals, uncoordinated and untrained (anyone could set up in practice as a 'psychoanalyst'), he saw the necessity of establishing criteria and certain qualifications if the Society were to be recognised by the medical profession as a legitimate branch of psychiatric medicine.

When Adrian and Karin approached him in 1919 as putative candidates it was a setback to be told that they must work for a medical degree concurrently with their analyses. Adrian was then thirty-six, Karin thirty; they would have reached their forties by the time they had qualified as psychoanalysts. What riled them was that James and Alix Strachey were allowed to practise as lay analysts, when James's attempt to read medicine at St Thomas's had foundered after six weeks. Their distinction was that they had had six months analysis with Freud which counted for more than a medical degree!

Getting a medical qualification is not taxing for anyone with a good brain, practical ability and a retentive memory, and Adrian had all three. Karin was handicapped by her deafness and here Adrian could be of service. She need not attend lectures; Adrian could retail them verbatim. She had difficulty in auscultating her patients, though some kind of ear-trumpet was devised for her.

Adrian hated his time at University College Hospital and after qualifying found it difficult to remember he was a doctor, though Karin enjoyed her medical training, in spite of her deafness. Without his medical degree Adrian could not have had his career as an army psychiatrist in World War II, nor attained his reputation as a valued member of the British Psychoanalytical Society. Psychologically his profession gave him stability and self-respect; he would never again be the man 'without an occupation', deprecated by Virginia. For Karin, whose interests included neurology and the management of psychotic patients in hospital, her degree was equally essential. Without it she would have been less respected during the six successful months she was to spend in America and would not have been invited to attend clinics and examine patients.

In 1919 they began their medical training at University College Hospital. James Glover analysed them both[53] from the end of 1919 till his death in 1926, when Adrian went to Ella Sharpe, Karin to Sylvia Payne. Both were elected associate members of the British Society in 1927.

In spite of her analysis Karin continued to have misgivings,

[53] Before long, the analysis of husband and wife concurrently by the same analyst would become unthinkable. (Freud himself was doubtful about attempting to treat both James and Alix Strachey, though it seemed to work in their case.) The reason may have been that there were so few trained practitioners in England.

though never about her work. She still suffered from an unfulfilled need for love and knowing she was loved. She still sought recognition, not just from her colleagues who admired her as a philosopher, but for herself, her whole personality. She still felt compelled to behave awkwardly, even brashly, in a way which alienated the very people from whom she most coveted friendship – Adrian's friends. She was not always oblivious to what other people felt or to her effect on them and she could be a reliable friend whose generosity of spirit warmed those with whom she felt at ease. But inwardly she felt herself to be a social failure and was continually turning over problems between Adrian and herself.

In such personal difficulties Adrian could be of no help to her. But he could be 'useful' (her term) simply by being there, by acting as interpreter when her hearing was particularly bad. During her medical training he was invaluable.

Only the deaf can appreciate the torment it must have been for her, eager to respond, apt in repartee. The temptation is to shut oneself off entirely. That she did not testifies to her courage and persistence, and no doubt partly explains her 'pushy' manner, specially when ill at ease. That she must often have been in pain counts for less than the barrier between herself and others. She could lip-read up to a point as the deaf instinctively learn to do. And her mother had sent her to America where she was taught by experts. One cause of her aversion to the Strachey family is understandable: they 'mumbled', nor did they take care to look at her face to face.

Karin wrote to her mother every two or three days. Perhaps to prove that the once-neglected daughter could claim the friendship of some of 'the best people' in their respective fields, there is some name-dropping in her letters. She sought out remarkable men and women for her own reassurance and no doubt to compensate for what she felt to be the rejection of Adrian's 'Bloomsbury' circle.

Just such a friend was William Rivers, neurologist, psychologist, physiologist of the sense organs, and anthropologist, all of which he regarded as different aspects of the same problem – the biological reaction of man to his environment and the fuller understanding of man's mind.[54] With his warmth, humanity and broad spectrum of interests coinciding with Karin's own, he was exactly the man to appeal to her.

In August 1919, having dispatched the children with Daisy, Ray and her children to Chilling, Karin and Adrian took a house in Cambridge, her spiritual home, primarily to attend a course of

[54] Lives of the Fellows of the Royal College of Physicians of London, 1826–1925.

lectures on psychology given by Rivers. On their return from Cambridge to Tanza Road Karin continued work on her book on Bergson and was further preoccupied with a paper to be given to the Aristotelian Society. She and Adrian never felt settled together; perhaps a move to Gordon Square would improve matters? It seemed that no. 50, still occupied by the army, would be vacated the following year. Later, in 1919, Adrian bought the lease, though it was to be some months before they moved in. Meanwhile Vanessa found room for them all at no. 41.

On February 13, Virginia noted in her diary that she had met Adrian at Duncan Grant's private view. 'Surveying the room with Adrian I thought him despondent, like a man aware of failure, and contrasting his life with those of his contemporaries. "How distinguished we all are!" I said. And then it came out – or did I imagine it all? – that he and K feel themselves isolated and like people who have been ploughed in some examination.'

Memory or not, her sisterly intuition was broadly correct. There was no real reason for Adrian's feeling of failure. However, he and Karin, like everyone else, were exhausted by five years of war and its aftermath. Adrian had been very ill, Karin sporadically unwell, their two small children had had serious illnesses, and now they were rebuilding their domestic life, a task for which neither of them was suited. They were starting out on a new, demanding career studying medicine and reading for their ultimate aim to become psychoanalysts; there was, too, the destabilising effect of their own analyses.

A deeper cause for Adrian's sense of failure was Karin's unhappiness; she was restless, perpetually tired and, like many another wife, blamed her husband for her dissatisfaction. The bond which had kept them together through the changes and disruption of war now fell away. They felt cut off from Adrian's Bloomsbury friends, but in this he was helpless. Karin was not altogether welcome and Adrian felt her rejection bitterly. We know from her letters to Mary Berenson that there were times when she became increasingly hostile to Adrian; she hardly mentions him, as though she alone met friends, carried on a social life and was on her own in the medical school. It was as though she was shouldering him aside, a necessary nuisance. Adrian's response, a chilly reserve, only exacerbated her irritation and despondency. Yet they could be seen walking affectionately hand in hand in the garden of Gordon Square, in thoughtful, amicable talk.

Apart from psychoanalysis they had one abiding interest in common – their love of the sea and sailing. From 1919 onwards they enjoyed sailing with Karin's uncle, Logan Pearsall Smith. At every opportunity they cruised with him and his one-man crew along the south coast. Now they looked for a boat for themselves. They found *Gadfly* which cost £150. Boats, houses, a car, operations – Karin had only to express a wish and quote the price for Mary and 'B.B.' to supply what was asked for. From time to time she dispatched a detailed run-down of her financial expenses, itemising even the smallest outlay, for their reassurance and to show that she was thoroughly practical about money matters. Bernard Berenson was by now extremely wealthy, his fame as a connoisseur of the arts unsurpassed in America. And, through Mary, he was generous. It would have been better if Karin and her sister Ray had been given a settled income; but, as we know, Mary wanted to have a hand in their lives.

Their visits to Chilling might have given Adrian and Karin an opportunity to be with Ann and Judith, often there in the summer with Ray and her two children, Barbara and Christopher. But they lost no time in dashing off to *Gadfly* on her mooring, setting sail and breasting the strong tides of the Solent. They made all the mistakes of impetuous beginners, gybing when they meant to go about, getting stuck on a sandbank, confused by the local 'double tides'. It was all 'tremendous fun', and the best possible relaxation.

As to the children, they still saw very little of them, either when they were with Ray or in Gordon Square. Karin was an affectionate mother when she was with them, and observed their development with some interest. The trouble was that her visits were sporadic and unpredictable: she would dash down to Ray's house, Copse Cottage near Haslemere, hug them, put them to bed and talk to them like adults, noting down Ann's thoughtful questions. Ann took her mother's muff to bed with her, and was ready to love her had she not been continuously frustrated by her absence, which she interpreted, as neglected children do, as being unloved and this, somehow, through her own fault. The complicated reaction to feeling unloved turns to hatred, as it did with Ann.

Adrian, like many fathers of his generation, hardly counted though he took them on his knee and drew pictures for them as his father had done. When Ann was taken to the pantomime 'Puss in Boots', he illustrated the story for her. As both children grew older he read to them. At birthday parties and at Christmas he played a

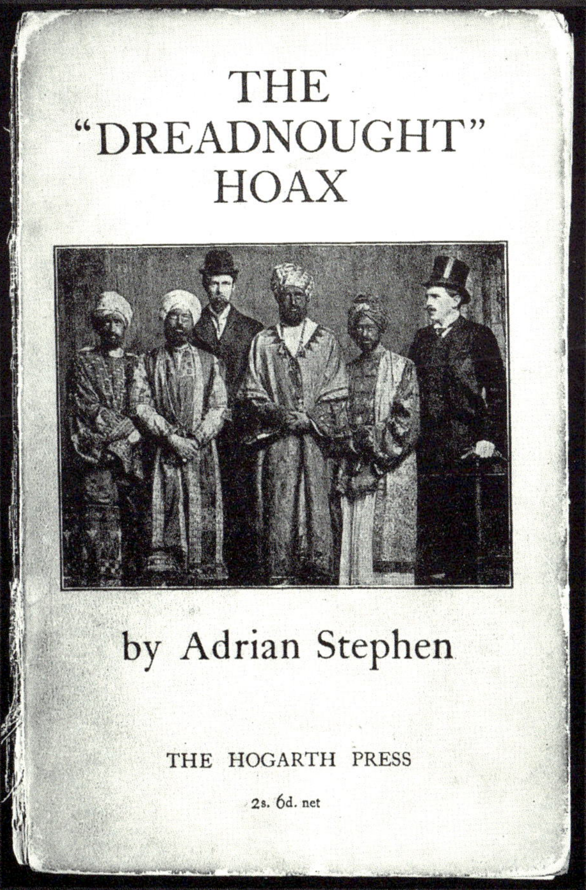

The cover of the first edition of Adrian's account of how they teased the Royal Navy. Adrian wears a bowler hat, as the interpreter, Horace Cole, his fellow hoaxer, is top-hatted. Duncan Grant on extreme left, Virginia Woolf next to Cole. The only crisis on HMS *Dreadnought* was when Duncan's beard nearly blew off and Adrian hurried him below. Adrian wrote that soon, 'It was hardly a question any longer of a hoax. We were almost acting the truth.'

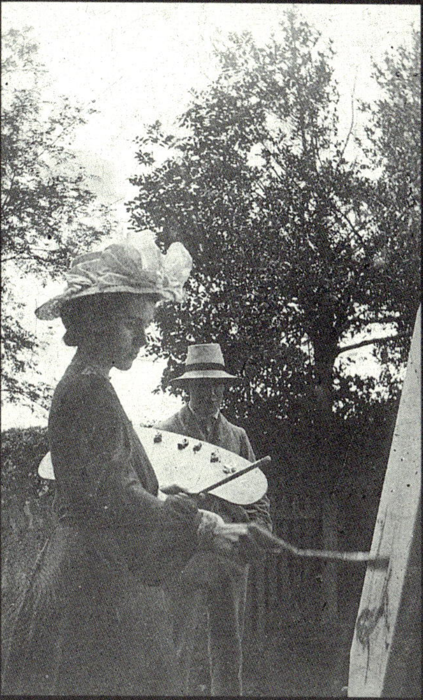

Vanessa paints at Fritham, 1903.

Clive Bell looks on as Vanessa cuts Lytton Strachey's hair, Asheham 1913.

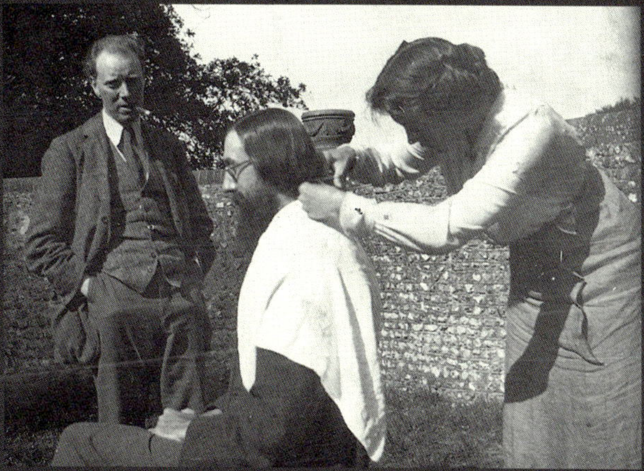

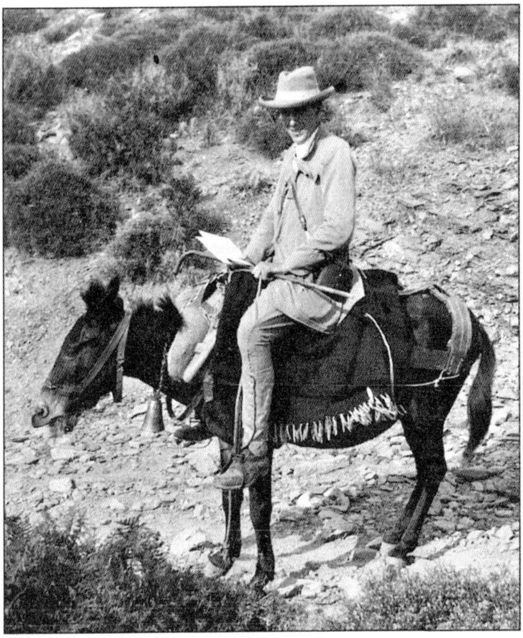

Thoby.

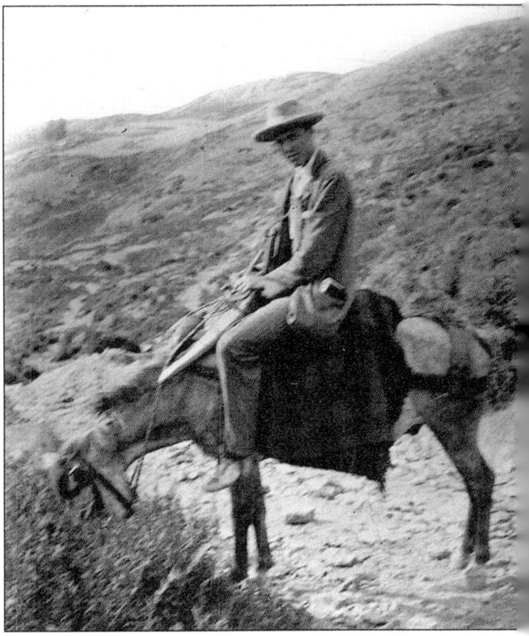

Adrian.

Greece, 1906. Thoby and Adrian went on what was then an adventurous journey, beginning by steamer in the Adriatic down the Dalmatian coast, landing at Cantano, whence they rode or drove through Montenegro to Athens. They went over the Peloponnesus, meeting Vanessa and Virginia at Olympia.

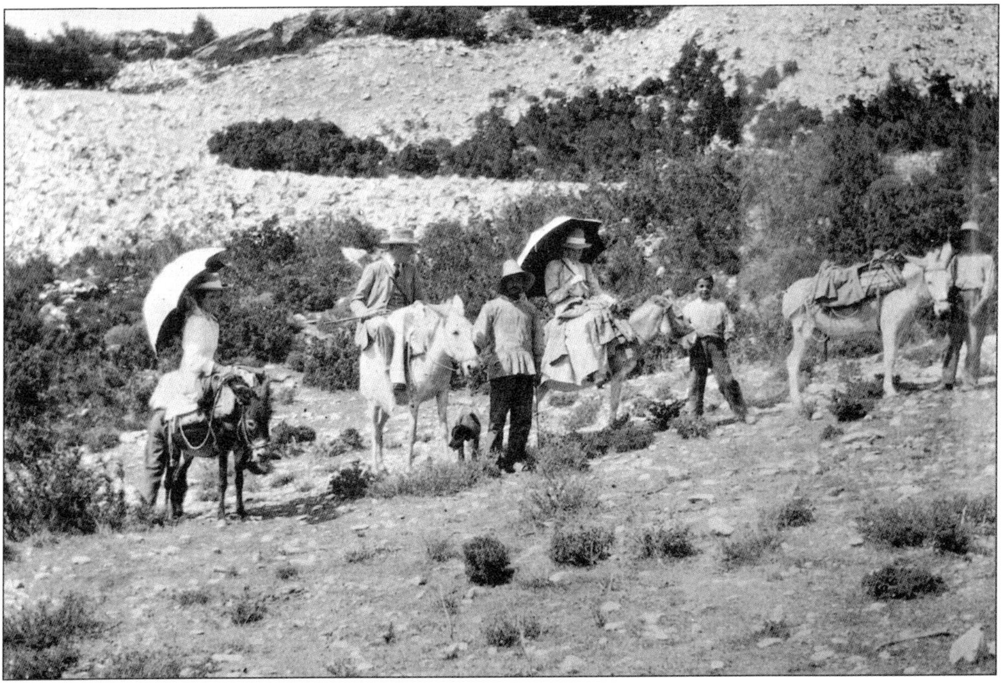

Mount Pentelicos, mounted left to right: Vanessa, Thoby, Virginia.

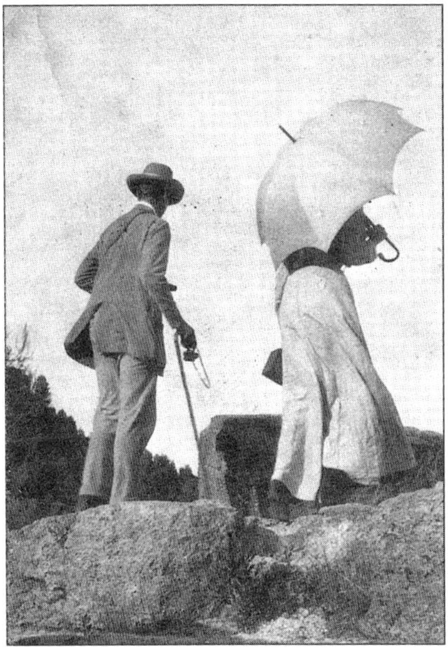

Thoby and Vanessa.

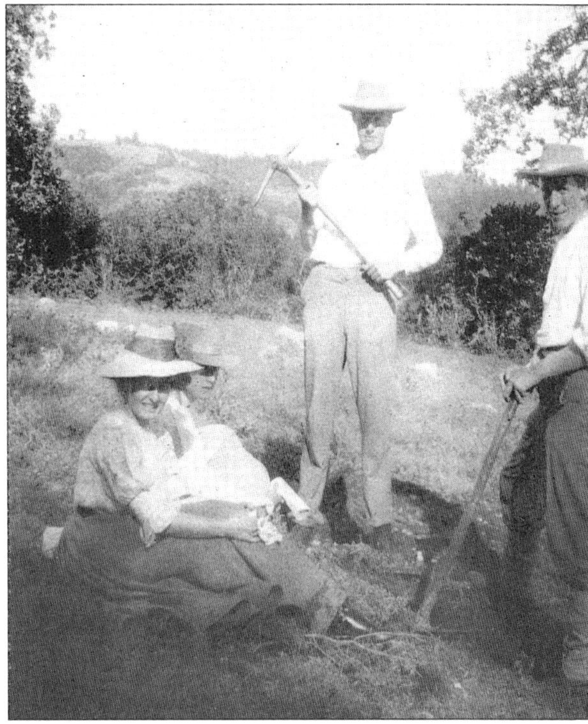

Virginia, Adrian and Thoby excavating.

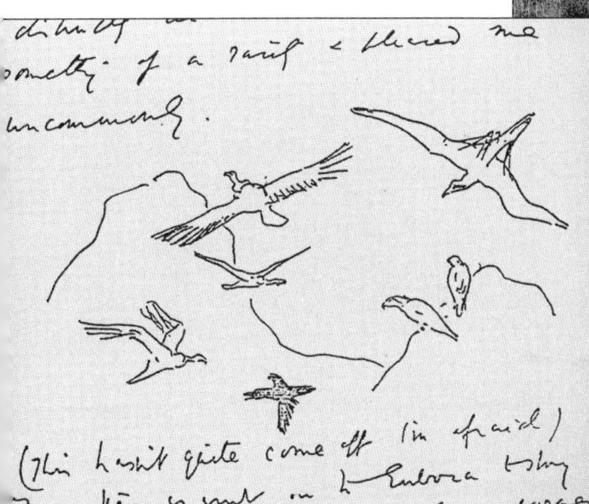

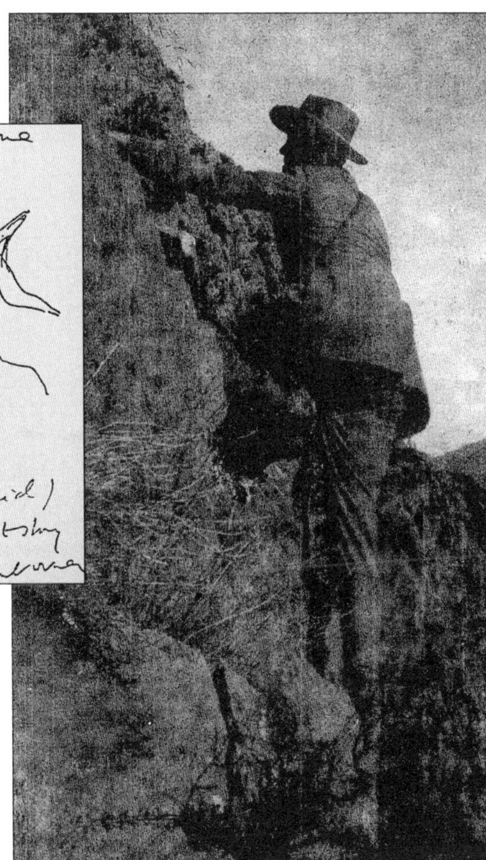

Thoby stalking eagles and his drawing of some of them in a letter to Clive Bell.

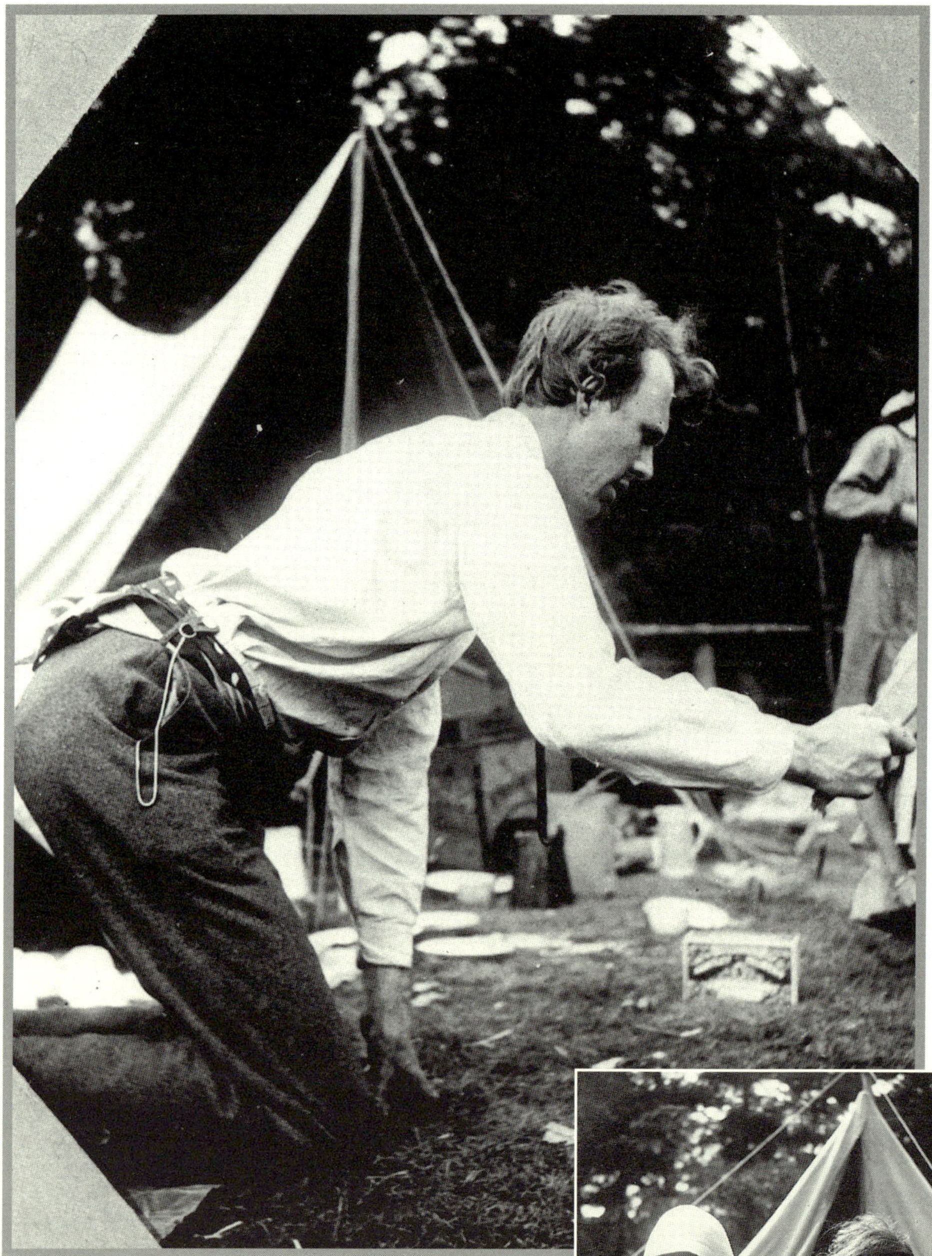

Adrian.

Camping at Brandon, 1913.
Among the campers were: the Olivier sisters, Maynard Keynes, Vanessa Bell, Duncan Grant, Roger Fry, Clive Bell and Molly MacCarthy.

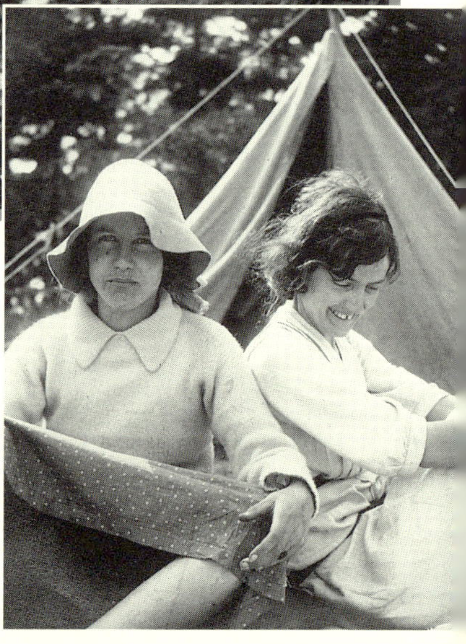

Noel and Marjorie Olivier.

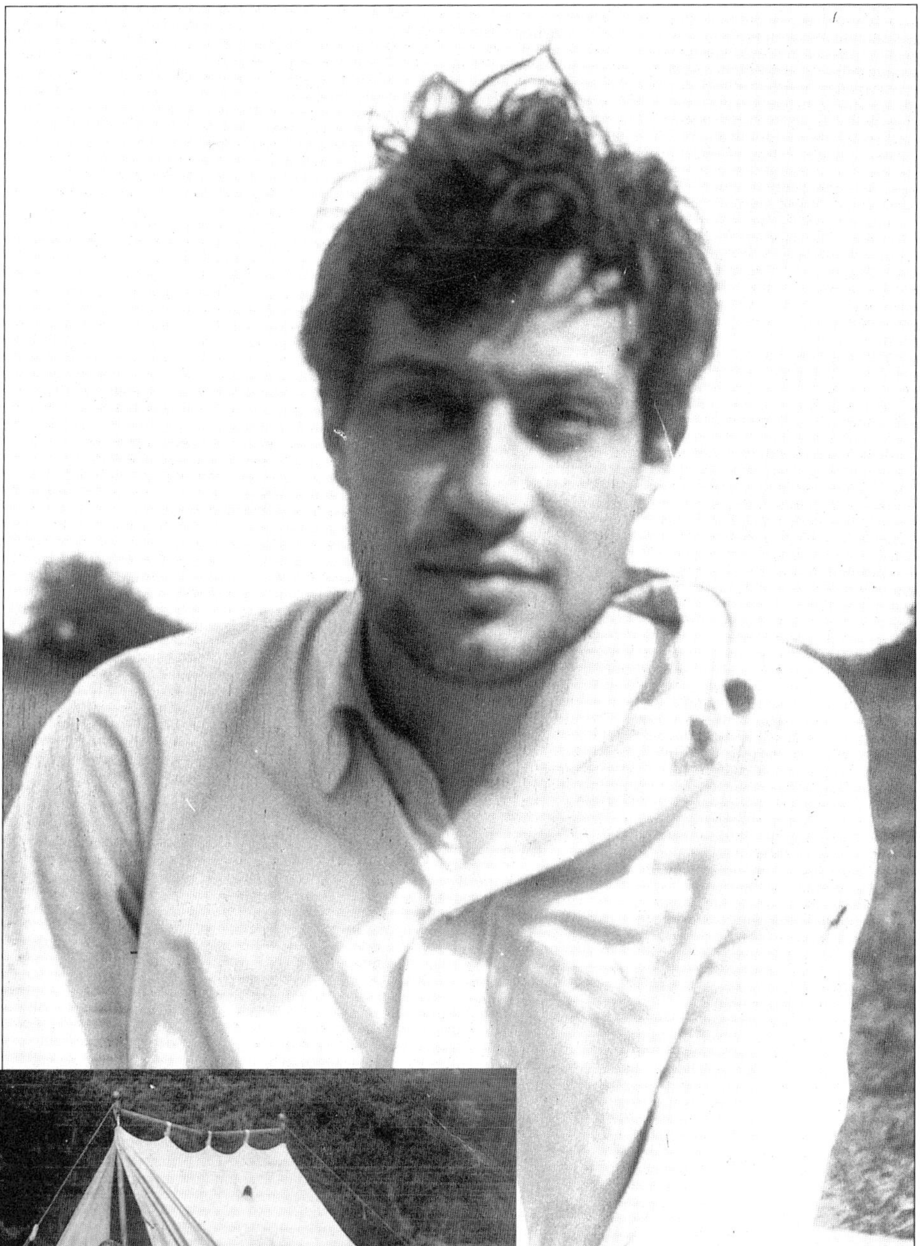

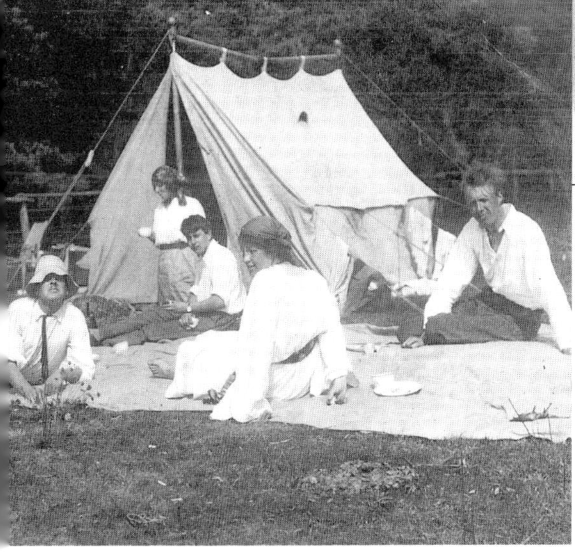

Duncan Grant.

Adrian on right. The two women are probably the Olivier sisters who were present: Noel wrote of Adrian (who was in love with her) 'I worked up an odious indignation against the good Adrian, not even to be calmed by his radiant beauty, as it appeared when he dined in his pyjamas . . . Later on I felt much more amiable.'

Karin, before her face had been disfigured after her operations for deafness which were, at best, only partially effective.

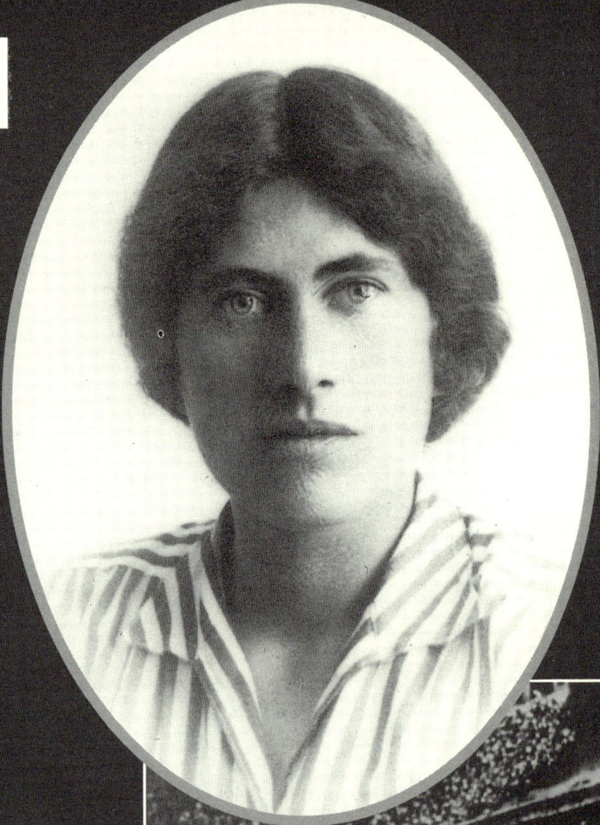

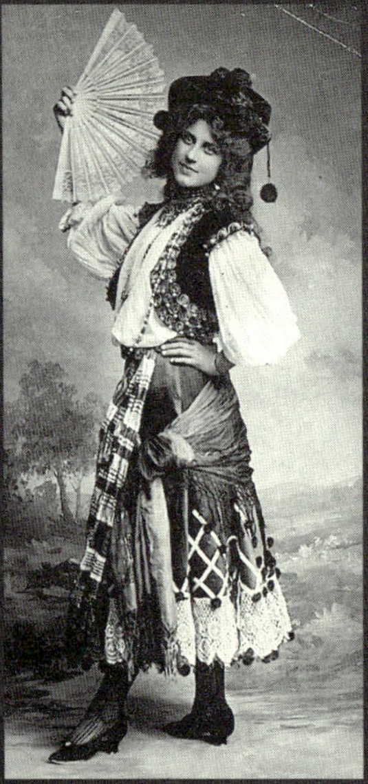

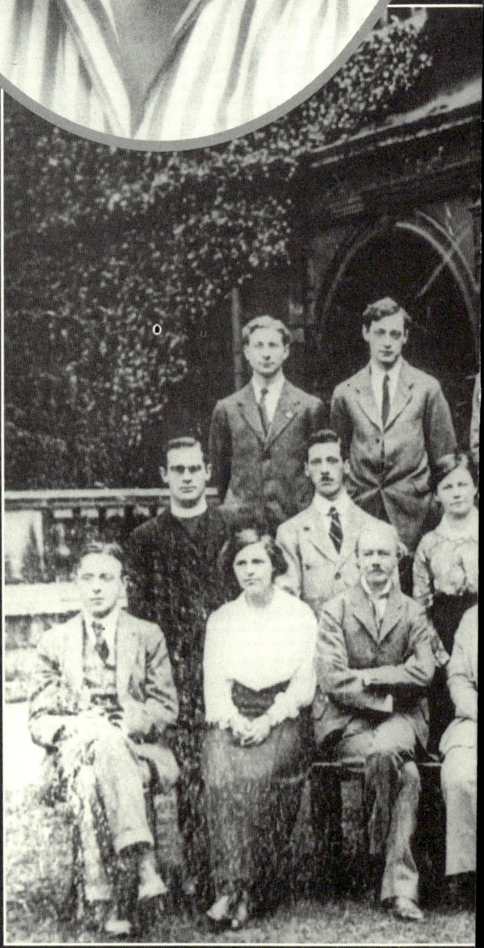

Above
Karin loved to wear fancy dress, here as Carmen.

Opposite top
Bertrand Russell's congratulatory letter on Karin's First-Class degree. He had insisted on being her tutor.

Right
Cambridge Moral Sciences Club, 1915. Karin is in front row, one from the right; Russell is fifth from the left. He wrote of Karin: 'She's a nice girl if only she were not so graceless.' G. E. Moore sits third from right in middle row; J. M. E. McTaggart, Hegelian philosopher and an Apostle, is on the far right, middle row, looking more than faintly disinterested; I. A. Richards is second from the left in the back row. (*Reproduced with permission of the Master and Scholars of Trinity College, Cambridge.*)

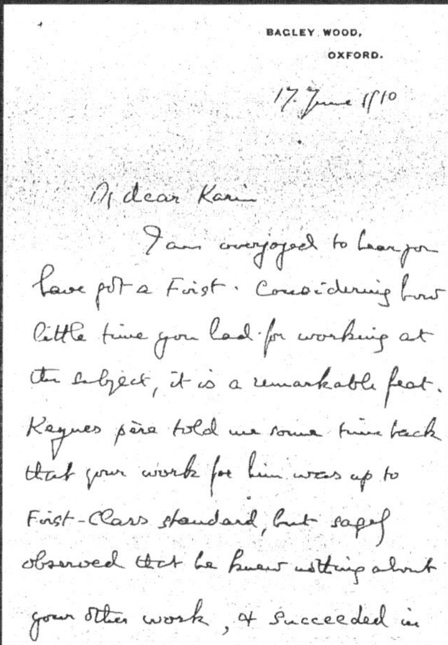
BAGLEY WOOD,
OXFORD.

17 June 1910

My dear Karin

I am overjoyed to hear you have got a First. Considering how little time you had for working at the subject, it is a remarkable feat. Keynes père told me some time back that your work for him was up to First-Class standard, but sagely observed that he knew nothing about your other work, & succeeded in

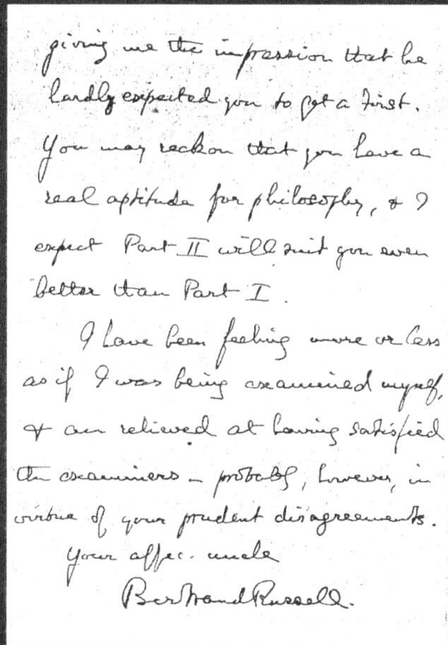
giving me the impression that he hardly expected you to get a First. You may reckon that you have a real aptitude for philosophy, & I expect Part II will suit you even better than Part I.

I have been feeling more or less as if I was being examined myself, & am relieved at having satisfied the examiners — probably, however, in virtue of your prudent disagreements.

Your affec. uncle

Bertrand Russell.

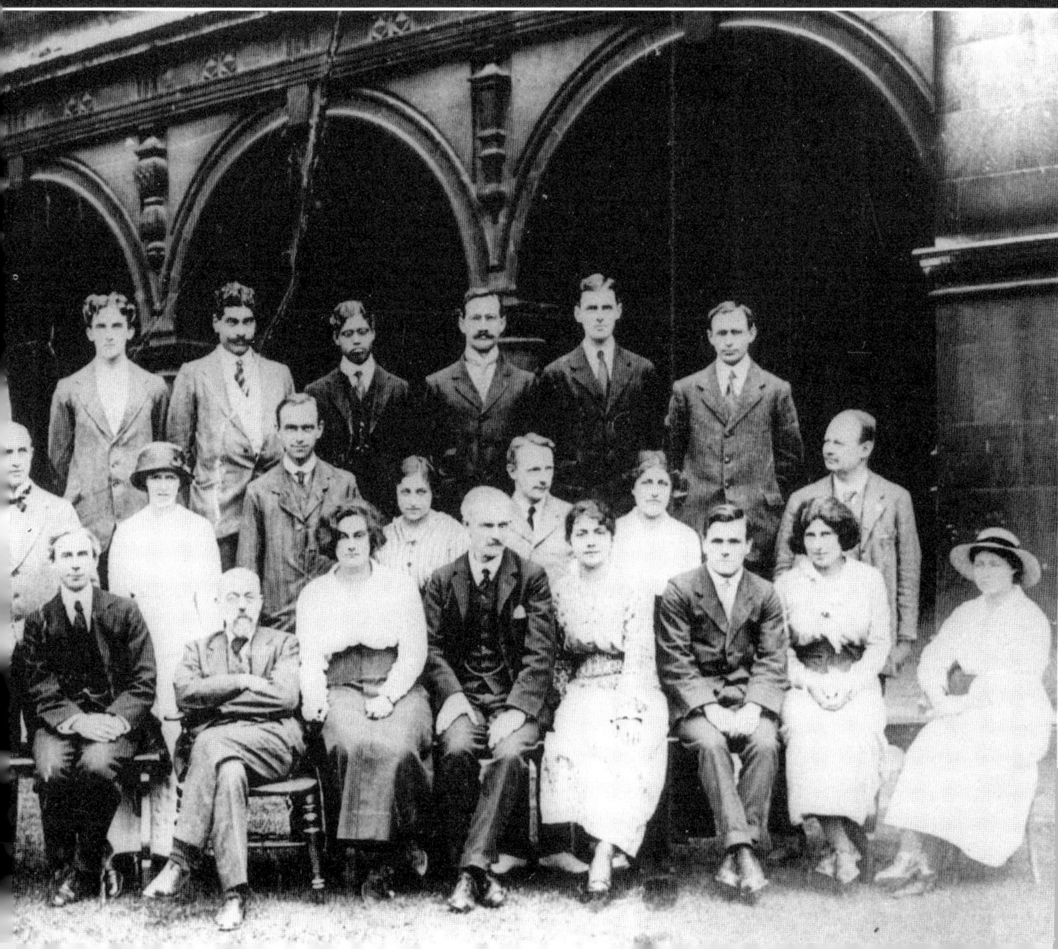

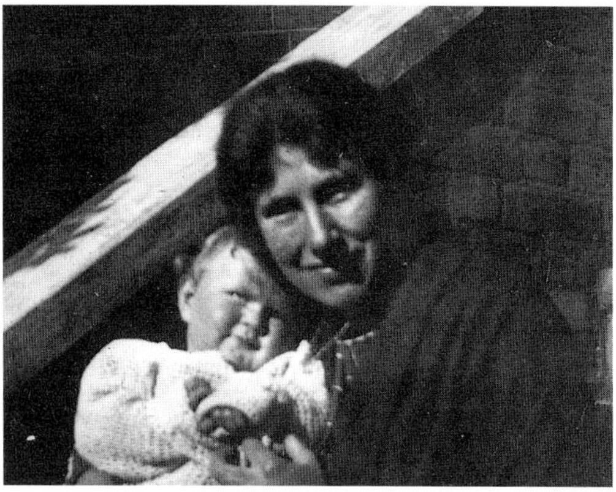

Karin and Judith. Karin always preferred Judith, Ann preferred her father to Karin.

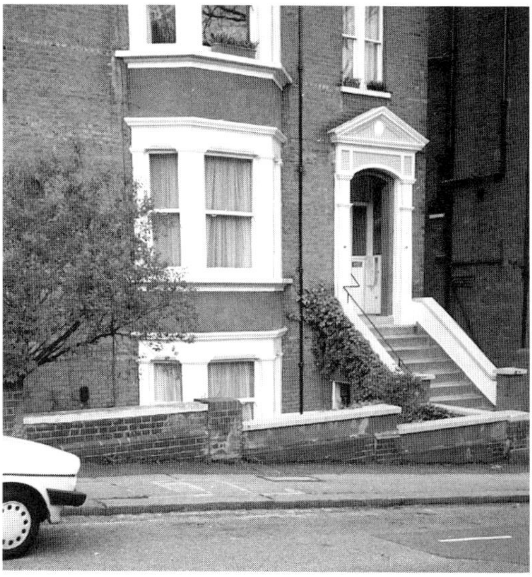

29 Tanza Road, London NW3 (photographed recently), where Adrian and Karin lived in 1916, six months after Ann was born. They almost invariably took unfurnished houses or flats no matter for how short a time.

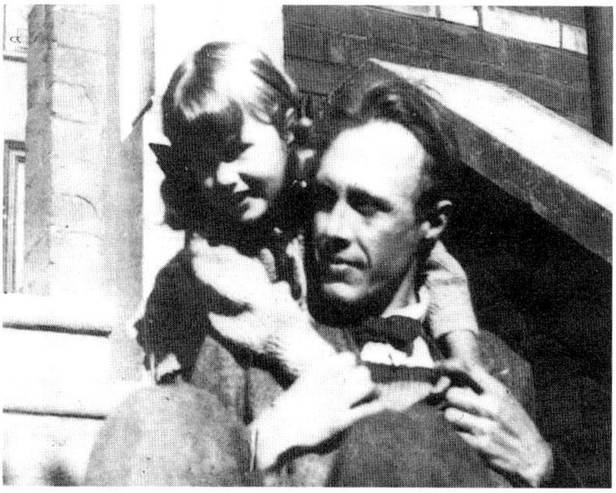

Adrian and Ann, Tanza Road, 1919. She is three.

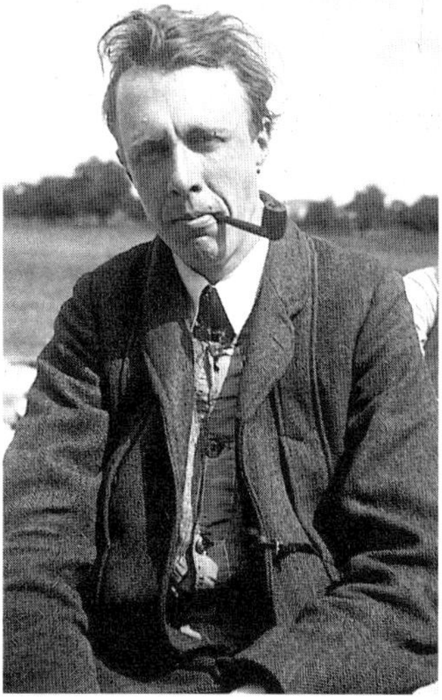

Adrian at the King's Head in the early 1920s. Both he and Karin went there whenever they could and they took up sailing seriously.

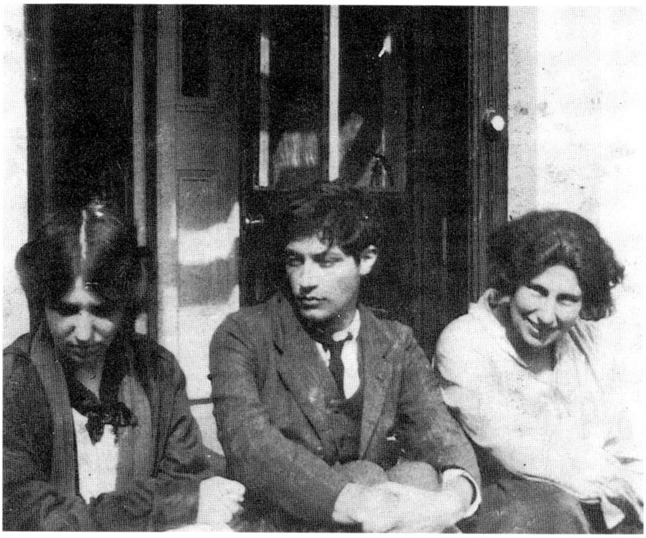

Hope Mirlees, Duncan Grant and Karin at Wilmington, 1915. Adrian was working at the UDC that year and wrote to Duncan: 'Hardly a day goes by now without a letter appearing over my name in some paper in London.'

father's part, acting charades, letting off fireworks. Once at least Adrian and Karin visited Copse Cottage together for a few days: 'Ann and Judith are very happy and Ann is extraordinarily pretty.'

By March 1920 they were all established in 50 Gordon Square. Vanessa moved from no. 46 and she and Clive and their family lived in the top half of no. 50 until she made her permanent home at Charleston. They were flanked by Lady Strachey and her family at no. 51. Alix Sargent-Florence and James Strachey lived at no. 41.

On May 1 Virginia wrote to Vanessa from Rodmell, the Woolfs' house in Sussex, that there had been 'a dreadful party' at Adrian's, mostly Berensons in full evening dress, 'hale and buxom and breezy . . . Aunt Lou was there and Hope Mirrlees. Karin made up her mind to show her spots – if that's the expression – I mean not to go in for art; so there was no nonsense, and Adrian in evening dress, but it's much better like that; and I am going to tea with her to see the children; and one of these days you will be surprised to find out how much nicer Karin is than anyone else.' But at other times she was distressed by signs of their unhappiness. She understood Karin's dismay, faced with the contradictions of Adrian's character. On the other hand Karin had begun to put him down, to belittle him in public. Quentin Bell remembers her saying scornfully, 'Adrian can be quite useful occasionally.'

Adrian vented his irritability chiefly on those he was attached to and lived with; on Virginia whom, in a brotherly selfish fashion, he loved, and Karin whom he needed and, in a way, cared for deeply. His friends were used to his barbed wit and cold withdrawal, alternating with open friendliness and concern.

A tragic occurrence showed Adrian at his best. In June 1920 Karin's Aunt Lou gave a party for Julia Strachey at no. 50. Virginia describes the incident and Frances Partridge who was there, corroborates her version.

> On the flat extension roof at the back there was a low parapet on which people sat. There were nightlights in coloured glass all round. A young man whom no-one knew, bent over to light his cigarette, overbalanced and fell over. Adrian, the only one to see him fall, got hold of a doctor who was there, went down and climbed into the area, examined the body, phoned for an ambulance etc. It was Adrian who traced his parents and broke the news of their son's death. He was quiet and practical throughout.[55]

[55] *Memories* by Frances Partridge, London, 1981.

Aunt Lou wanted to go on with the party, as though nothing untoward had happened. 'She was a Panglossian,' Frances Partridge commented. Her insensitivity caused frequent distress, particularly to Julia Strachey, brought up in her care.

(In 1941 when we first met, Adrian himself told me the story, at least the bare facts, omitting his own part in it.

'How awful it must have been! What an appalling shock!'

'Not really. We didn't know him,' he replied drily.

At the time I felt chilled. Most people would have made a proper story out of it, the drama, the details. I was not used to the plain truth.)

He may have taken comfort from being back among friends, in the place where, if anywhere, he belonged. But there was a price to pay: the very closeness of the houses, the daily intercourse between their inhabitants, favoured gossip. The talk often centred on Adrian and Karin, on her growing animosity, his increased waspishness. Adrian was said to be broken up by his analysis – but would be put together in time. His analyst was reported as saying, 'His tragedy is that he can't enjoy life with zest.' This last Karin told Virginia when she came to tea with Ann. Virginia wrote, 'Ann is like him, pale, lanky, sensitive with long cold fingers I know so well.' Ann was old enough to take in what was being discussed. Thus early on, the child may have formed the gloomy view she afterwards took of her father's temperament. 'The truth is', Virginia continued, 'Karin does not fertilise the sunk places in Adrian. Neither did I.' Sometimes when she went to tea with Ann and Judith, Karin was there. Once she found them all at tea in the nursery with Sophia Farrell, the devoted family servant who took charge during Vanessa's absence. Quentin and Julian played with Ann in the garden. Ann tall, with long fair hair, already promising to be a beauty, became friends with Julian and it was a loss to her when they moved to Sussex. She and Judith were not often asked to Charleston.

It is true, I think, that Adrian needed family life, wanted to be a family man, as Virginia wrote in her diary. She thought Karin had given him this fulfilment, a sense of being 'like ordinary people'. But Karin's fulfilment lay elsewhere with scope for her brilliant brain and the companionship and deserved admiration of her peers. As for helping to create a family, she herself had never known loving parents; she had been unloved by her mother, her aunt and grandmother who brought her up.

Not that she didn't try: they went to a lost dogs' home and

bought a mongrel, 'mostly retriever. We have been longing for a dog to complete the family. I feel we make up a perfect domestic unit.'

The year was occupied with work and sailing. 'Adrian beat me in the zoology exam –3rd in a class of 50. I beat him in physics, coming second.' During the vacation they moved restlessly from place to place – to Cassis where they were 'looking for boats' – though they already had one. They took a house again in Cambridge for Rivers's lectures on psychopathology.

In May 1921 Karin completed her book on Bergson and sent it off to the Cambridge University Press, enclosing letters from Whitehead and Bergson himself.

In their medical examinations Karin got Firsts in three out of four subjects, Adrian got straight Seconds. In June they had their last weekend on the boat before going again to Cambridge, renting 16 St John Street once more for the Rivers lectures where Duncan Grant visited them.

While still in Cambridge, Karin hoped to get to Chilling to see the children. 'I'm sure Judith is going to be a darling, funny, and excited and full of energy.' But this hope was deferred. In those days analysts habitually went abroad for their summer break followed by their patients so that their analysis could continue. This year James Glover went to Berlin. Adrian was to go there first while Karin awaited her turn, in Austria. Before leaving they made a brief excursion to the East Coast to see a house Karin had heard of in Tolleshunt D'Arcy, near Maldon, the first indication of a move that was to bring them all happiness.

Adrian in Berlin with James Glover wrote that he had 'benefited enormously from his analysis and has never before in his life been so happy'. He picked up Karin at Kitzbühl so that they could have a few days together before resuming their analysis with Glover. 'I am very much excited', Karin wrote rather surprisingly, 'at seeing the darling [Adrian] so soon.' They went on to Vienna where they heard Freud lecture.

Back in Gordon Square in October, Adrian's analysis was still going well. 'He came back bubbling with high spirits – a rare state for him but he is promised it is quite a usual one if he can work off his complexes. He could not tell me what had happened as we are not supposed to; but he feels as if an ancient weight is now beginning to roll off his spirits.'

It was at about this juncture that 'J.F.' makes an appearance as a friend and medical man. Dr John Freeman was a bacteriologist at St Mary's Hospital, Paddington, specialising in asthma and hay fever. He was also an immunologist, well in advance of his time. He had transferred a sample from Ann's infected ear to her sound one to immunise it. Tall, good-looking and sympathetic, he was fond of women and had a steady relationship with a woman outside his marriage which his wife, Violet, tolerated *faute de mieux*. He was just the man to appeal to Karin, and from 1922 onwards was a frequent visitor to the house.

What were his feelings for her? Probably he felt a certain attraction as well as compassion for this brilliant, impetuous woman with her flashing blue eyes and dark gypsy complexion, and an unsatisfied longing for a romantic lover. Karin fell passionately in love with him, describing their relationship as 'an affair'.

By December the united family hoped for by Adrian and Karin was somewhat awry. Adrian was feeling the strain of his analysis, hard work and poor lectures at UCH. Ann was in bed with a high temperature.

The beginning of 1922 was not promising. Ann still had a high temperature and swollen glands. Her doctor said that her tonsils must come out. Karin stayed with her in the nursing home the night before the operation. Ann was becoming more and more like her father in looks and in temperament. And it may be partly due to this that Karin, after a while, favoured Judith, a Costelloe, dark and inexhaustibly energetic.

Once made aware of Ann's increasing unhappiness, Karin provided for her what proved to be a lasting benefit: she arranged for her analysis with Ella Sharpe. After a fortnight Miss Sharpe wrote, 'Ann's imagination is the most delightful and delicate and original' that she has come across in a small child. 'But she must be gently handled or she shrinks up.'

At this time (February 1922) Virginia Woolf recorded in her diary:

> Adrian is so happy & genial that I am really pleased. I don't want to make him out a failure even. An unambitious man, with good brains, money, wife and children is, I dare say, the most fortunate of us all. He need not protect himself by any illusions. He sees things as they are. He is humorous, contented; free to enjoy without envy or uneasiness. 'Oh well,' he said talking of his medical career, 'it's something to

> do. It's easier now to go on than to stop,' he said. He has his ya(t)cht, & as the years pass, he will ripen into a delightful father. Moreover, like the whole family, he has this distinguished, cool point of view, which always makes him good company, & admits him to any society – if he wished for any society, which needless to say, he doesn't.

In August Adrian and Karin again went to Berlin to continue their analysis, and stayed on till September to attend the Seventh International Psycho-Analytical Congress. Since they were not yet members, they were not allowed to attend the banquet, nor the official business. But they met many English members in the meeting hall. Joan Riviere was there, John Rickman, Ernest Jones and James and Edward Glover, and other seasoned members. They had a talk with James Strachey whose analysis with Freud was in train. And there were the illustrious Berliners, Sachs and Eitingon and Abraham with his protégée, the young Melanie Klein. Freud himself came with his daughter Anna, and all the Viennese analysts. The scene was just what Karin needed to dispel depression.

But their return to England saw a fresh onset of her restless dissatisfaction.

'I must get away,' she complained, 'I must have a place of my own where I can be alone, or entertain my friends.' Her affair with J.F. was sporadic. Karin had planned to meet him in Austria; but J.F. cried off.

How did Adrian fare, living with Karin's changes of mood? He read Freud in the original German without difficulty. He doggedly continued his hospital training, hating every moment of it, unlike Karin who enjoyed the active part, working in casualty, in the theatre or delivering babies in the district, though, since Adrian could not be there, her hearing was a handicap.

The solution for them both, though long delayed, was to be Landermere and the King's Head, at the head of the Hamford Water (Arthur Ransome's *Secret Water*). They had viewed several houses; then, after leaving the main road, bumping along a rough track between fields lately harvested and studded with Cambridge elms, they came to Landermere. Before them lay a great expanse of water-meadows and salt marshes, islands and mud-flats threaded with shining tracks, creeks broadening out to wider and wider stretches of water, and beyond, the sea, misty blue in a September haze smudged by a steamer's smoke. Arching over all the East

Anglian sky poured down light as though reflecting the ocean.

The King's Head, a tall, broad, sizeable building of mellow brick, rose up almost from the water's edge. It had been a public house when barges tied up at the wharf to unload their cargoes before the coming of the railway killed their trade. A weather-boarding addition on a smaller scale had been built on to the landward side, warmer and more comfortable. But what captured their imagination surely was the lofty principal room, 'the long room', as it came to be called, that ran the length of the main part of the house. Two of its tall windows looked east over the saltings, another westward over the garden, a long grassy expanse running alongside the creek to an overgrown orchard with plum trees and bushy shrubs that hid the privy. Four greengage trees grew almost at the water's edge; their fruit never failed to ripen and split, ready to eat.

Karin was careful to write to the Berensons that she was not acting on impulse, but taking thought, consulting surveyors, etc., details on which Adrian, by training and nature, was well qualified to advise her. And perhaps he did. But in her prevailing mood she wrote exclusively about my house, my children, my friends.

She finally rented the property, early in 1924, for £650 per annum fully furnished, having agreed to pay for repairs. 'At any time I might buy it for £650.' (She bought it in 1932 for £1,500.) But before renting it she went down often, as though it was already hers. 'I think about it a lot.' It served to distract her though it did not dispel her depression.

'There is only a small scrap of land with it, just enough to make a garden, and a stall for a pony and a coach-house for a ponycart.' There was a dilapidated wooden structure, which housed first a donkey and later a pony and cart. She even considered installing central heating! The King's Head could never have been centrally heated with its steps and corkscrew stairs and crannies consequent upon the joining of the old and the new buildings, let alone the two bedrooms over the long room, reached by a lethal staircase some forty or fifty feet high.

With her plans for Landermere, the occasional visits of J.F., the distraction of work at UCH and her analysis, which she already began to anticipate leading to openings in her special interests – neurology and the treatment of psychotic patients – Karin, for the greater part of 1923, seemed happier. The children, though still prone to fall ill, were more often at home with Daisy in the nursery, and attended a school run by Marjorie Strachey in the square. Ann, it is true, was still unaccountably depressed, in spite of Karin's efforts to find out why. Probably Ann was puzzled by her parents' uncertain relationship and saddened by her father's unhappiness. Her parents were seen walking as usual in the gardens in deep conversation – or, it may be guessed, Karin talked and Adrian listened. Whatever their difficulties – and their Gordon Square neighbours were aware of imponderable uncertainties, Karin sometimes showing signs of frenzied despair, Adrian at his most taciturn – yet they seemed, by November 1923, to have settled matters between themselves.

They were seen everywhere, demonstratively fond of one another. So it was a surprise to everyone when it was announced that they were going to separate. Vanessa rang Virginia with the news when they were in the middle of dinner. In her diary Virginia wrote: 'You could have knocked me down with a feather . . . the devoted and inseparable couple! . . . I was overcome by hearing they had been unhappy for years.' Two days later she met Adrian in the bathroom at no. 46. 'I kissed his hand and he burst into tears. 'It's an agony!' he cried. So we went upstairs holding hands . . . We walked to the bus and he told me it had never been right – almost, but never quite right. They hadn't quarrelled.'

Vanessa and Clive agreed that 'Karin did it more than he did. She felt all I used to feel: the snub; the rebuke; the fastidiousness; his lethargy.'

That was a sister's view of their marital breakdown, and probably Karin had felt something of what Virginia had suffered. But as we know from Karin's diary of 1913–15, there were other factors. It may be guessed from the same source that these two needed each other but did not love each other – unpropitious ground for a successful union.

On November 27 Karin wrote to her mother: 'Of course you would understand and sympathise. . . . But the really bad unhappiness is over for both of us. . . . We shouldn't have hung on for so long . . . I shouldn't have had the courage to break it up at all without analysis. I haven't the faintest doubt that a complete separation was essential, at any rate for a time, no *modus vivendi* would have given us the feeling that we could and must tackle life afresh without depending on or hampering each other. Glover entirely approves.' Here she seems coolly practical, and probably with reason. But did she have to turn him out of his own house so light-heartedly? 'We have found a charming flat for him in Mecklenburgh Square.' She and the children would be able to go on living in no. 50 if she practised economy. The Bells still rented the top-floor flat. She launches into one of her complicated financial exercises, the gist of which was that she would have to pay Adrian rent. And he would have the rent from the Bells; but until he had begun to earn as an analyst she couldn't allow him to contribute to the maintenance of the children. She ends with the conclusion that she will have a little over £1,000 a year, Adrian about £340 – 'poor soul!' (he had rather more than that – over £500).

In this crisis Adrian psychologically needed her more than she needed him. His near-prostration may be accounted for partially by his early experience: one more desertion casting him into the black hole of misery and guilt after his mother's death, worsened by Thoby's death ('The wrong man died'). There was too his pride; we know the importance he attached to marriage; he had failed as husband and father. Then there was the Stephen emphasis on success, the disgrace of failure, about which Virginia was specially concerned for him. In February 1922 she had written to Vanessa, 'I have seen Adrian – perfectly charming detached from Karin; and really a success in his own way.' And in November he had spoken to her Woman's Co-operative Society on psychoanalysis which he did well. In any case their separation was complicated by their having to meet during the day. They were still medical students, and Karin needed him. But in the evenings he was banished to his lonely flat.

A detached, amused but sympathetic observer was Lydia Lopokova, a well-known ballet dancer whose career was coming to an end. Maynard Keynes, her beloved companion, had arranged for her to rent rooms at Alix and James's house, 41 Gordon Square, while he was obliged to spend most of his time at King's College, Cambridge.

On November 15, 1923, she wrote in her charming version of the language: 'Adrian and Karin fluctuate in conversation. Karin wants affairs physically speaking. . . . Up to now they spend the day together on psychoanalysis. In the evening they go to the cinema.'

In April 1924 'Adrian started his solitary life in another square spending the day as usual with Karin, but the evenings and nights are such a misery for him that he nearly committed suicide, the fact is that he longs for Karin and Karin looks for other dimensions, and prefers Adrian not to be with her most of the time.'

'Dimensions' is a good word; true Karin wanted a lover and the brief 'affair' with J.F. partly satisfied her craving for romance, though it was probably enhanced by her wish-fulfilment. But she certainly needed to spread her wings, get away from husband and family and pursue her working life elsewhere for a while.

Adrian, as he had done before, adapted himself to new conditions. And life in Gordon Square had advantages. He was among friends and could be in and out of their houses on familiar terms. He was asked to parties. He even read Virginia's latest book, *Mrs Dalloway*, published in 1925.

Adrian spoke with his customary teasing irony and, in this case, ingratitude, of his sister-in-law, Ray Strachey, who had so often fielded his children when crisis threatened. She practically brought them up in their pre-school years. She was, he said, 'one of our dangerous feminists that should be destroyed, that she always wore trousers in the country, and no doubt too many combinations.'

Other friends came into Adrian's life about this time in 1926. Frances and Ralph Partridge joined the Gordon Square contingent.

> A new friend was Adrian Stephen whose immensely tall lean figure was often to be seen loping round Gordon Square, sometimes accompanied by his clever, deaf wife, Karin. I was reminded of him as I wrote about our railway accident and the shouts of 'Doctor!', because he once told me that on the very day he gained his medical degree (in order to practise psychoanalysis) he went to the cinema, and it so happened that an urgent voice from the door interrupted the film with a cry of 'Is there a doctor in the house?' 'Like a fool I said "yes",' said Adrian. 'However' and here he gave his characteristic laugh – long, melodious and ironical, 'there wasn't much I could do. I was confronted by a man who had been run over – and his head cut off!' Adrian's striking face with its rather haunted expression might have been that of an eminent philosopher or scientist. In fact he liked girls, enjoyed parties, and had a very good sense of humour.[56]

In conversation, Quentin Bell spoke warmly of Adrian at this time. He 'has often been described as sad and gloomy. He liked fun and laughter, light-hearted companions, parties. It depended a little on who he was with.' Quentin was warmly appreciative of Frances: she was, he said, just right for him and brought out his light-hearted side.

[56] Ibid.

Karin, for her part, was making the most of her partial freedom. She writes to her mother in January that she and Adrian are 'adjusting to the new situation and I feel great hope that all will end happily. Don't be afraid that I shall get melancholy.'

Her letters during 1923 to 1924 refer often to 'J.F.' with whom she is growing closer in 'intimacy'. His confident ebullience consorted well with Karin's character and they were close companions for a time. As to 'intimacy', the extent of this seems doubtful. Doctors have been known to risk sexual relations with patients; they can't be 'struck off' unless a complaint is made. The doubt is whether Karin, physically, either wanted copulation or would have been sexually attractive to men. Her 'gracelessness', regretted by Bertrand Russell, did not lessen with age. Her figure remained curiously lumpish, clumsy and, like her taste in clothes, uncoordinated; and her eagerness on the dance floor, transposed into sexual approaches, could have made her intimidating.

When to such speculations is added her fantasiste exaggerations, the probability is against the consummation of her 'affair'. In April, 1924, J.F. 'broke it off', though he continued to treat Ann and Judith, and was welcomed as a friend. Karin loved him and spoke of him to the end of her life.

In her diary, February 9, 1924, Virginia wrote: 'Karin has been confiding. Adrian wants to come back. She wants life. I don't altogether like her, kicking up her heels, yet see her point; and respect her conscience, for she has A. on her mind. He sits alone in Mecklenburgh Square. "It's the quality you Stephens have", she said. "It's the real thing like an American with a Sheraton table."'

In September Karin suffered a further check to her plans: her cook, Lottie, and Adrian both had temperatures. 'I couldn't let Adrian fall by the wayside and have given him a bed here. He really doesn't depress me at the moment at all: I feel as though this whole time was an interregnum and didn't count and I just must live through it till I get rid of the hospital and put my house in order.' She felt that she had to continue with Adrian till 'this rush is over' – presumably their coming examinations at UCH are on her mind – 'not only out of kindness to him; he is the only person who can do my ear for me . . . it needs doing so often . . . at least once every day and often more . . . Meanwhile I constantly have to ask Adrian in order to keep up with things I want to do . . . It is an awful coil from which I can't seem to escape while I go on at the Hospital. My hearing makes it impossible for me to get on by myself.' J.F.'s breaking off 'the affair' and his retreat to Devon with Violet precipitated a bout of depression. She wrote that she feared a breakdown and that Adrian was necessary to her, however 'ludicrous'.

Christmas celebrations were muted by Judith's severe illness: J.F. took a sample of her blood; she proved to have paratyphoid fever. Day and night nurses were engaged, and Ann fetched back from the nursing home where she had had an operation on her ear. It was at this juncture that Adrian and Karin planned to go away for the weekend, scandalising their friends. Ray forbade them to move. But Karin went off leaving Adrian who, nevertheless, decamped on the Sunday, leaving Daisy in charge of the household.

On December 31, 1924 Karin went to the King's Head, having taken it for the week. Eventually she decided to take it on a permanent basis, unfurnished, an arrangement that was to continue till she bought it in 1932.

The first summer at the King's Head went well. Arthur Ransome lent them his boat, *Racundra*, till they found one of their own. Friends were invited every weekend. A German girl, Charlotte, was engaged, partly as 'governess', partly as general help. One of their earlier visitors was Duncan Grant in 1925.

> *Wednesday, the King's Head*
> Dearest Nessa, Here I am after my first day's visit to Karin, so I suppose I must give you some account of it. To begin with, it is a strange tumble-down sort of house but certainly rather attractive. All our bedrooms lead out of one another and there is one long sitting room which is really rather charming with windows on 3 sides & rather extraordinary views over the mud flats. It is extraordinarily remote only a few cottages near & a few trees round the house. Last night there was a howling wind & I should think, it might get appallingly desolate in winter but luckily today has been fine & rather mild & the country is the sort I find sympathetic. The house trees & estuary might have come out of an early Constable with children & old boat builders & all the rest of it. In a part of his ramshackle house lives an elderly man & his wife & 4 children who play all the time with Ann & Judy. Lottie cooks all the food in the kitchen & also there is a young German female called Charlotte who is rather nice & looks after the children does all the odd jobs & apparently for no money. The noise & turmoil are terrific during the

> day. This morning I did a little sketching. This afternoon the Stephens took me for a sail down the estuary to an island where we took our tea, coming back & tacking against a strong wind unluckily the peak halyard broke the sails came rattling down & the mizzen nearly struck me a bad whack on the head. Carry as Clive says is not at all a bad girl as you know but *il y a des gouffres d'indelicatesse!* Yesterday she did a thing even Gumbo [Marjorie Strachey] might have hesitated to do – she offered me some gin & then pulled up her skirt & wiped the cup on her drawers! All of course in the best spirit of camaraderie – but I had to refuse the gin.
>
> The children seem to me to have become mere raga-muffins but I dare say it is no bad thing & they seem perfectly happy and barbarian.

Adrian and Karin had both qualified as doctors in 1925, and in the same year he became a member of the British Psychoanalytical Society. Karin gained her associate membership in 1927. There were now signs that they were coming closer. On May 19, 1926, Virginia wrote to Vanessa, 'Adrian and Karin are inseparable and are re-arranging the house [no. 50] beds now being only one wall off [next door].'

For the children, the King's Head held untold bliss. Naked they slid down mud banks like seals at low tide. They padded barefoot along the seawall and squelched over the saltings to the Cardinal's Hard; here there was a channel where boats could be moored, ready for an early departure when the tide allowed. The place was lonely, but not forbidding; with not a human habitation in sight, nor mankind except for a sail or two moving far off through the islands; Hamford Water and its wide stretch of marshland and water meadows was a world of its own. For those of us who knew Adrian and the place, there was an affinity between them.

That summer, then, promised to be happier for them all. But the autumn was overshadowed by the prospect of an operation on Karin's ear which, if successful, would improve her hearing. She was unwilling to risk an operation with an uncertain outcome. But Adrian and Mary advised her to have it done. The result was disastrous; a nerve was severed leaving her with a disfigurement down one side of her face as though she had had a stroke. She struggled with shock and depression for weeks, supported by Adrian. 'About Adrian I will write to you more later. We have had some serious talks and I am deeply touched and grateful for his love and constancy and understanding.'

'Elli',[57] their new GP, advised convalescence in a warm climate. Karin's better ear was blocked and it 'will not come right till Adrian charms it away'. She went to Bermuda, meeting 'Mrs Somerset Maugham',[58] bound for Nassau.

Karin returned home in April, and wrote to Mary on June 1: 'We have just got frightfully good news. Adrian has passed his MB BS examination and now has an absolutely first-class qualification. He has been working for it the last six months but did not want to say anything about it in case he failed.' In August she wrote: 'I am glad to say that Adrian has got a job as Clinical Assistant at the Maudsley. He has already been given a patient of his own to treat! The work is unpaid but it is a beginning . . . He is frightfully keen to earn money and his failure to get paid work has depressed him very much.' (This last is for Bernard's benefit.) It is unlikely that Adrian was so upset – it was all part of his training; but her frequent apologies in the same vein suggest that there were rumblings at I Tatti as to Adrian's inability in the past to contribute much to his family income.

And in January 1927, when they were both accepted as associate members of the British Psychoanalytical Society, with considerable courage for she was sensitive about her facial disfigurement, Karin set sail for America. This was a great success. She visited Boston, New York, Philadelphia and Baltimore and renewed contact with her American relations. More important for her were the numerous introductions to eminent practitioners in the fields of neurology, psychiatry and other allied disciplines, disciplines which were always to distract her from straight analytical theory. Her visits to various hospitals and discussions with capable and innovative colleagues stimulated and delighted her, and she formed valuable friendships. She fleetingly considered looking for a post in America, and described this time as a 'dream interlude'.

[57] No doubt Elli (Dr Francis Eleanor) Rendel, daughter of Lytton Strachey's eldest sister, also Virginia Woolf's and other Bloomsburys' GP.

[58] Syrie Maugham, fashionable interior decorator, wife of the writer.

15

THE KING'S HEAD

That summer after Karin's return was the pattern for one sailing season after another, and indeed for all seasons, for Karin enjoyed wintry expeditions. For Ann and Judith, secure in their mutual attachment, the King's Head was a source of freedom and delight. Here their offhand upbringing mattered less, if at all. Grown-ups might shake their heads; but much of what seems to adults shocking neglect, is not felt as such by children. Their aunt, Virginia, was appalled to hear that their parents, cruising off the south coast, had sent for them to join the boat at Newhaven. They had no money; but trekking across country, thumbing lifts and foraging for food seemed no more to Ann and Judith, aged about ten and twelve, than an entertaining challenge. They cared for the donkey and pony and drove in the cart over the countryside together.

Amabel Williams-Ellis in her book, *All Stracheys are Cousins*, recounts an incident which illustrates Stephen insouciance at sea. She and her husband, Clough, had jointly hired a boat with them and were tacking as they made passage out of the Medway, the channel being marked by huge towering black buoys numbered in white. She and Clough were in the cabin preparing breakfast and could hear Adrian and Karin in the cockpit:

> 'I think with the tide as it is we should leave No. 4 to starboard.'
> 'Plenty of room with Plover's draught either way.'
> 'But what about the wind on this tack?'
> 'Yes, she does make a good deal of leeway.'
>
> This placid debate goes on for several minutes when we hear a loud bang and feel a shiver run through the boat,

> almost sending the full boiling coffee-pot out of Clough's hands and the bacon out of the pan I am holding on the stove . . . as expected we see Plover scraping along the black side of the towering No. 4 buoy as the tide races past.

Ann and Judith were a striking feature of the King's Head. Ann, already above average height, unkempt, wild, but 'beautiful and fair', Judith, dark, handsome, more approachable. Ann's friendship with her cousin, Julian Bell, continued; he came to the King's Head several times, though she seldom returned his visits to Charleston where Judith was more frequently seen, probably because she invited herself. Ann's reticence prevented her from making a move which might have been welcome. They were often happily on their own during school holidays; for their parents, except for analytic holidays and longer seasonal international congresses, had to sandwich weekends between patients.

The years between 1919, when they began their training, and 1927, when Adrian and Karin became associate members, had seen enormous changes in the British Psychoanalytical Society. When it was founded in 1919, one of Ernest Jones's first concerns was to ensure that new members were genuinely interested in becoming psychoanalysts. In the early days a number of people from widely different fields and disparate interests had become associates. Men and women who were attracted by Freud's writings but, without undergoing analysis, took what they understood to be his concepts and adapted them in a distorted form to fit their own preoccupations.

During this period the *International Journal of Psychoanalysis* was founded (1920). The Institute of Psychoanalysis was set up in 1924 and while the translation of Freud's books was under way, largely through the energy and influence of John Rickman, the Hogarth Press became joint publishers with the Institute of *The Psychoanalytical Library*. In 1926 a clinic was established for the benefit of 'needy patients'. 96 Gloucester Place became the headquarters of the Institute, the British Society, the London Clinic of Psychoanalysis till 1950 when the Institute moved into 63 New Cavendish Street.[59]

It was during this period – 1919 to 1929 – that Ernest Jones put so much effort into establishing Freudian psychoanalysis as a legitimate part of psychiatry. After lengthy meetings of a special committee of the British Medical Association, including Jones himself, it recommended that the claims of 'Freud and his followers to the

[59] Pearl King, *Psychoanalysis International: A Guide to Psychoanalysis Throughout the World*

use of the term (psychoanalysis) are just and must be respected.' It defined psychoanalysis as 'the technique devised by Freud, who first used the term,[60] and the theory which he has built upon his work'. Jones thus gained for psychoanalysis recognition of its differentiation from other forms of psychotherapy.[61]

While Jones could be rigorous in establishing discipline among his colleagues, he was essentially liberal and forward-looking when considering the general direction and future of the international psychoanalytical movement, and his experience internationally had taught him that the unity and close identity of the theoretical conclusions, technique and practice of the early analysts was no longer possible if psychoanalysis was to remain a science and not degenerate into a dogmatic theology.[62] He favoured the pragmatic approach which was shared by so many of his British colleagues, including Adrian Stephen.

Adrian and Karin were at the Salzburg conference in 1924 when Jones chaired a symposium on 'The Relation of Analytic Technique to Analytic Theory'. 'In all these fundamental matters . . . both of theory and practice, my plea would be essentially for moderation and balance, rejecting nothing that experience has shown to be useful, while ever expectant of further increase in our knowledge and power.' This accorded with Adrian's temperament and beliefs, less closely with Karin's divergent interests which kept her darting between disciplines.

Before long Jones's belief in the importance of open-mindedness and new developments was to be tested. There was already a growing interest in child analysis in England: Nina Searle and Sylvia Payne had written papers on theoretical and practical problems of the subject. Now, largely through Alix Strachey, who had become a close friend of Melanie Klein while they were both in analysis with Karl Abraham in Berlin, and had gradually become convinced by her conceptual and practical advances in the analysis of children, Jones invited her to give a course of six lectures in London. Miss Searle offered her house in Gordon Street, adjoining Gordon Square, and there in 1925 Melanie Klein burst upon the British analytical scene.

Although some work had been done on children over the age of six, almost nothing was known about the mental life of younger children: Freud's conclusions were drawn from the analysis of

60 It was Coleridge who first used the term 'psychoanalysis' – *The Notebooks of Samuel Taylor Coleridge*, Vol. II (1905).

61 Pearl King, ibid.

62 Ibid.

adults. Klein's detailed knowledge of early development enabled her to confirm directly what Freud had inferred from adult material. Her unmodified Freudian techniques to child analysis – she would give neither advice, reassurance, nor any educational guidance – aroused intense opposition among some, and equal support by others; also her findings were found shocking and therefore unbelievable, even by those who had come to accept Freud's views on child sexuality. But the wide acceptance and tolerance of her views which permeated the British movement led her to settle in London in 1926.

As Ernest Jones writes in his preface to *Contributions to Psychoanalysis* (Klein, 1948), 'Cries began to be raised that in the views she vehemently presented she was "going too far", which I think simply meant she was going too fast. The trouble was she was pursuing [her views and methods of work] with a novel rigour and consistent recklessness that evoked in some members at first uneasiness and gradually an intense opposition.'

Adrian and Karin for a time supported her. At a Society banquet Virginia and Leonard Woolf sat at their table with Melanie Klein and Roger Money-Kyrle, a veteran of the Royal Flying Corps and one of her champions. Virginia was persuaded to ask her to dine. She came, but the evening was not a success; they didn't take to her. The arrival of Melanie Klein and the controversy over her findings were to result, some twelve years later, in an event of crucial importance to the Society and to Adrian and Karin.

When Karin returned from a second visit to America in March 1929, she found Adrian established at no. 51. In correspondence with Mary Berenson, the unrealistic idea of Adrian moving away altogether evaporated. It is doubtful in any case whether Karin could have let him go, so deeply entwined were they in their need for one another. The present plan suited her well enough, giving her freedom to live more or less as she chose, but close enough for daily meetings and walks round the gardens in amicable discussion.

Ann and Judith were, before long, sent to day-schools, Ann to Queen's College, Harley Street, Judith to St Paul's. Ann, preferring her father to her mother, spent most of the day with Adrian, who occupied two floors at no. 51.[63] She remembers that they were looked after by a Mrs Mansfield who had been housekeeper to the unfortunate 'Tussie', Karl Marx's daughter. Talk between father and

[63] Barbara Halpern Strachey, an authority on her family, questions whether Adrian ever occupied part of no. 51. But Ann's recollection is clear and there are letters from Adrian to Mary Berenson which confirm it.

daughter at lunch was light-hearted. Adrian, like most people at the time, was mindlessly anti-Semitic. Jews were legitimately thought 'funny'. They ate a kind of melon called 'Honey-dew', referred to jokingly as 'Honey Jew'. A friend of Judith's remembers him, when reading aloud, as being specially good at imitating Jews. This generally held view involved a curious split in the minds of Gentiles for whom Jews were close friends. Their hostility surfaced when they thought of Jews *en masse*, outsiders, too clever by half, an amorphous, threatening lot – 'The Chosen People', 'a certain race'. This digression is relevant because Adrian wrote a paper, 'Anti-Semitism', still in manuscript, unpublished as far as I know, and undated, though clearly prompted by the rise of Nazism and perhaps by the arrival of analysts from Vienna and Berlin, in which he analyses in some depth the causes of the sickness.

As Ann remembers, her parents in the Thirties were chiefly occupied with work; with establishing themselves in the Society, now firmly organised, largely through the efforts of Ernest Jones, with a growing nucleus of able men and women, lay analysts and psychiatrists, among them John Rickman, Edward and James Glover, Joan Riviere, Alix and James Strachey, Ella Sharpe, Sylvia Payne, Barbara Low and Melanie Klein. The Stephens were preoccupied with getting patients, in attending meetings, and, Karin specially, in contributing papers.

Some of these papers were written for the medical section of the *British Journal of Psychology*, founded to give members of diverse psychological interests – psychologists, psychoanalysts, psychotherapists, anthropologists and neurologists like W. R. Rivers – a meeting-place for discussion and the exchange of ideas. John Rickman was their president. He was, and remains, one of the outstanding figures in the British psychoanalytical movement. He was a Quaker, and he had seen service in World War I with the Society of Friends' ambulance unit in France. He brought to psychoanalysis that mixture of good sense, practical ability and a capacity to tolerate and work with people of differing beliefs and persuasions which characterise the Friends.

And it is perhaps because of the freedom to try out and feel their feet in their new, exacting profession that led the Stephens to contribute papers to the Psychological Society's journal. Some were kept by Karin and found among her papers after her death, suggesting that they had some significance for her. Adrian's style and approach were very different from Karin's. Quentin Bell defines the Stephen way of writing:

> They . . . all had some gift, some pleasure in the use of the English language. But they wrote like men who are used to presenting an argument, who make that argument plain but forcible. . . . Their minds are formed to receive facts and when once they have a fact so clearly stated that they can take it in their hands, turn it this way and that . . . they are content.

Adrian read *On Defining Psychoanalysis* before the medical section of the British Psychological Society on February 25, 1931. His choice of subject was no less bold than Karin's lectures on psychosomatic medicine. He writes like a true Stephen, but with his individual humour. He loved teasing; beginning by teasing at the subject then teasing his listeners as an introduction to his serious purpose. He leads them along a false trail, then disabuses them of common false assumptions about the practice of psychoanalysis. He continues by turning the subject this way and that, including the analyst's part as well as the patient's.

> My next illustration will perhaps seem far-fetched, it is that of making friends with a strange dog, let us say a savage watch-dog chained to a kennel. If gone about in the right way this is not usually a difficult task, though there are dogs with whom one would not want to make the experiment, just as there are patients whom one would try not to analyse. A good way, I think of approaching such an animal is just to stand quite quietly within the radius of activity allowed him by his chain, and to hold out one's hand. Beyond this, one must make no demonstration of either friendliness or hostility. At first of course, one is received with a volley of barks and the dog may fly at one and even snap, though more often he retreats into his kennel or gets on the top of it to bark from there. By merely staying quite still, showing neither fear nor favour, one can usually achieve success. The outbursts of hostility gradually subside, and the creature comes gingerly forward. He is still intensely suspicious, of course, and the slightest movement may reawaken his antagonism, but, if one stays quite still and lets him sniff one's hand at his leisure, the trick so to say is usually done.

He wrote one other paper for the British Psychological Society, 'Impotence' (1935), a contribution to a symposium on 'Nullity and

Impotence' held jointly with the Medico-Legal Society. It begins:

> I have been asked tonight to give an account of impotence from the psychoanalytical point of view, and it is none of my business to say anything about the law. I take it that an analyst has two main interests in the subject. As a physician he tries to cure impotence, and as a psychoanalyst he tries to understand its origin. But I shall confine my remarks to the question of origins, for this does not seem the moment to consider analytic technique.

The paper ends:

> And now I have spoken long enough, but before I finish I would say that I have not attempted to put forward original views. Every analyst could add a great deal more than I have left unsaid, and would perhaps make small corrections here and there, but I believe that on the whole every analyst would agree that as far as it goes what I have said is what is generally accepted.
>
> I can only thank Heaven that I have not got to propose any remedies for the legal situation. I rather think I know what sort of remedies I should propose if I had to propose any, but I can leave that in more expert hands.

The Stephens used no. 50, and for a short time, part of no. 41, Alix Strachey's house, as their consulting rooms. But Ernest Jones emphasised the importance of a 'good address' for their private patients, and in 1930, Yvonne Kapp, who was referred to Adrian by Alix Strachey, began her analysis with him in Welbeck Street. Shortly afterwards he, followed by Karin, took consulting rooms at 141 Harley Street.

Yvonne Kapp was married to Edward Kapp, the artist.[64] She herself was a writer using the name 'Yvonne Cloud'. She first came to Adrian 'completely out of kilter', owing to the break-up of her marriage. Her early impression of Adrian as an analyst was that he was somewhat 'God-like, rather remote'. He didn't, as she remembers, say very much or offer interpretations; she did most of the talking. She was sufficiently involved in the analytic situation to go

[64] Edward Kapp, an artist of considerable talent, will be remembered chiefly for his drawings, many of which are in the British Museum which commissioned twenty-five lithographic portraits by him of the delegates to the Council of the League of Nations.

through the early stage of intense resentment, anger and hostility. The analysis was broken off in 1932–3. She began again with him in 1937, this time in York Terrace, Regent's Park, the Stephens' home until the beginning of World War II.

During the resumption of her analysis Adrian was more active, made more interpretations. While maintaining the accepted analytic conventions he came out with responses that surprised and pleased her. For instance, he 'commended her new preoccupation with politics as a healthy sign', and said 'Good' when she told him about an affair which promised stability 'if not much else'. Yvonne agreed that during her second analysis she herself was more mature. She was extremely hard up, with a child to support; but she managed to pay, this being an essential part of analytical treatment. It typifies his kind-heartedness and idiosyncrasy that after a session he gave her half a crown for a meal! The analysis was again broken off in 1939 because the Czech Refugee Fund she worked for, a Government subsidised organisation ('Blood money!' she interjected forcibly during our talk) was being evacuated. During World War II she and Adrian became friends and occasionally met for dinner when they were both passing through London. 'One of his disarming traits was his readiness to declare how boring his nearest and dearest could be.'

Another patient of Adrian's was Wyn Henderson, who moved into Gordon Square in 1930. Wyn was a colourful, salient figure during the late Twenties and Thirties, with a large circle of friends, among them writers, artists, musicians and analysts, and she gave famous parties. Everything about Wyn was on a grand scale, her generosity, her friendship, her impulsive decisions – her analysis had to be broken off because, to quote her daughter, 'She left London rather abruptly to run a hotel called "The Lobster Pot" in Cornwall.' Even her sporadic abandonment of her three children had a fine, sweeping nonchalance. Susan, her daughter, first met Adrian when she was about fifteen and confined for six months in a fever hospital. Hearing of this through his patient, Wyn, Adrian visited her.

> He was so tall, so thin, wearing, in London, a navy-blue suit and black socks with brown shoes. I felt rather over-awed as he stood looking down on me from his great height. A small nurse kept jumping up at him, trying to robe him in a white gown, hood and face-mask. He sat down and was gentle and

> really charming. When I recovered, he said he would arrange for me to meet his daughter, Judith, who was the same age.[65]

He was as good as his word and she was invited to dinner at no.50. It must have been during one of Karin's absences, for Adrian was in control, and enjoying his rôle as father of the family. Before Susan's arrival he threatened to cut off Judith's allowance if she didn't tidy her room. (Ann, it was rumoured, kept rabbits in her room.) When Susan rang the bell, she found Judith at the foot of the stairs, holding the hand of a baby baboon, lent to them by their scientist friend, Solly Zuckerman. Their dinner was cooked by Grace, Vanessa's cook, lent for the occasion in the happy Stephen/Bell custom of swapping their servants, who never seemed to mind.

Judith invited Susan for the weekend at the King's Head. They met Adrian at Liverpool Street Station. Wyn, having told Susan (or 'Binkie', her hated nickname) to 'be good and impress Adrian', the young girl kept up an erudite discussion with her friend about Erasmus. At their journey's end Adrian, aware that he was meant to be impressed, said, 'Thank you, Binkie, for the intelligent, sustained conversation.'

The weekend was thoroughly enjoyable. They sailed – Adrian, she thought, 'rather inexpertly' – and in the evenings sat round a log fire while he read them S. S. Vandyne and Edgar Allan Poe making them as 'frightening as possible', acting each character. He frightened her so much that Judith had to accompany her down the garden to the privy. The two slept in the barn in bunk beds with the donkey – a great comfort.

When Wyn Henderson left Gordon Square Susan was at boarding school and her elder brother was in Manchester working for the *Manchester Guardian.* There was nowhere for her second brother, Nigel, to sleep. He worked during the day restoring pictures for the National Gallery and slept in Karin's waiting-room. She and Adrian grew fond of him; he took the place of the son they had longed for, and they rejoiced when he married Judith.[66]

Susan has another memory of Adrian. She was ill in bed at no. 47 when her 'schizophrenic grand-mother' came down threatening

[65] Susan Watson, extract from her diary.

[66] Judith appears hardly at all in the narrative, chiefly because she died long before this book was thought of. Also because we knew her much less well than Ann. However, during a day's sail not long before she died, we talked about her parents. She liked her mother better than her father, about whom she was dismissive. In her appearance, and with her formidable intelligence, she resembled Karin, though not in her nature. Judith was tolerant, friendly, and generally likeable.

suicide and left the house. Susan rang up her mother at work. Wyn came home; her grandmother returned in a strange state not knowing where she had been. Wyn, alarmed, fetched Adrian from no. 51 and he took over and had the grandmother removed to a mental hospital.

During the years of his partial banishment Adrian, according to Virginia, alternated between various moods. On March 27 she noted, 'Our set at Nessa's last night, was hardly at its best. L [Leonard] and Adrian silent and satirical.' But, in June 1927, 'Adrian came to tea on Sunday and fairly sparkled. Even his analysis will be over this year. At the age of 43 he will be educated and ready to start life. . . . We Stephens mature late.' In February 1927 Adrian had written to Vanessa from 50 Gordon Square discussing the sale of 22 Hyde Park Gate, which was let. Leonard suggested £7,000 as a good price for it. 'Will you let me have your views?'

> I hope everything is all right with you & that Duncan is well again. I have absolutely no news. I am living in the ground floor front room & go to the Maudsley every day & don't manage to see very many people outside the hospital. Maisie's disease has taken a turn for the worse & as she is in consequence not allowed out at night at all I don't get much chance of seeing her.

The identity of Maisie has not been traced but there is a suggestion that Adrian was attempting to console himself in Karin's absence in America by a passing affair.

But in May 1931 Virginia was writing of a more serious attachment. Adrian had fallen in love with Doris Chapman, intriguing but mystifying his friends. She was a painter, showed at the Wertheim Gallery, but was otherwise undistinguished. She was found to be dull, unappealing.

Susan Watson remembers that she appeared at Wyn Henderson's parties. She was about twenty-seven, long-legged, reasonably good-looking except for a curious, hooked nose, attractive and sexy. (Frances Partridge agrees with Susan, except for the sex appeal.)

Virginia wonders at Adrian's dwelling on the past 'when there is his present and his future all round him: D.C. to wit, and Karin coming in late, predacious, struggling, never amenable or comforting as poor woman no doubt she knows: deaf, twisted, gnarled, short, stockish – baffled yet still she comes. All these cold elements of a party not mingling . . . We meet James and Alix at the door. Come and dine, says James . . . I think to keep hold of Lytton . . . Adrian sepulchral, polite, emaciated, elongated, scientific. . . . We evaporate at 11.30: courteously thanked for coming by Adrian. Question what pleasure these parties give. Some, presumably, or these singular figures wouldn't coagulate.'

But Adrian's party is evidence of the way his friends loyally 'coagulate' round him at a time of stress.

The affair with Doris Chapman, as far as is known the most serious he had after his marriage, lasted about a year, from 1931 to 1932. She was ambitious; she needed money. She married a rich man, considerably older than her, a Mr Keiller of Keiller's marmalade, and they lived in Eaton Square, Belgravia.

In July Adrian wrote twice to Vanessa. The affair was tailing off.

> Of course you had to go away. You have been an enormous help to me this summer and so has Duncan & I certainly shall turn up at Charleston if I get in one of my wild fits but I hope I shan't. I have a little more hope again of getting on satisfactory terms with Doris again. She came to my party last night but very late & I am afraid I was in consequence rather a bad host. . . . The party broke up rather early but she stayed to the end & I saw her back to her flat – and then she asked me to come in for a strictly limited time & have tea. We just sat quietly & talked about things in general till 2.00 & then I left her. She says she can't come for a country walk on Sunday but would like to come to lunch and also to dinner on Tuesday. She is going away on Thursday having let her flat so that will be the last I shall see of her for the summer.
>
> The latest development in my plans is that I may be going to take over Lytton's rooms & use them as living & consulting rooms – keeping a brass plate somewhere in Harley St for purposes of consultation & so on . . . I am afraid I have upset Duncan rather badly – perhaps you a bit too – I just couldn't help it.

The emotional disturbance of the episode with Doris Chapman did not interrupt his analytic work. In 1927 he and Karin had become clinical assistants to the clinic attached to the Institute where patients who could not afford the fee for private analysis were treated. In October 1932 Adrian and Karin were appointed to the public lecture subcommittee with Rickman, Yates and Barbara Low. In 1930 he had given two papers to the Society: 'The Rôle of Homosexuality in Transference' and 'Sleep as a Transitory Symptom Formation: A Case where Sleep Became a Constant Defence'. (In recalling this, he said that he, too, tended to doze off!)

In 1933 Adrian gave six public lectures on 'Psychoanalytic Theory', chaired by Rickman. These lectures followed Karin's. She gave seven public lectures: 'Clinical Studies of Neurotic Patients'.

Nor was Adrian's social life much disrupted. He continued to see friends, to dine out, sometimes with Karin, sometimes on his own. In June 1933, on the evening of an Apostles dinner attended by Leonard, he dined with Virginia. Friends came in during the evening but sister and brother continued to reminisce about their childhood; their father, 'was he utterly bad?' 'He had friends,' Adrian said.

Later in 1934 Virginia was preoccupied, as she so often was, with Adrian and his marriage.

> Yesterday, just as we had done tea, Adrian's gaunt form appeared; Karin's tousled shape, grown very thick and large. Her inferiority takes the form of praising Adrian. 'Clever old Adrian!' she exclaims if he bowls a good bowl (on the Woolfs' bowling green at Rodmell). This is a way of saying – what? My marriage is not so bad after all? He remains perfectly unmoved, quiet, sensible; I suppose curiously immature, though able to go through all the actions perfectly, of a grown man, father, husband.

Another view of Adrian appears in Antonia White's diary in June 1933: 'I dined with Adrian last night and was happy with him – though I have never known a person so nervous and guilty.' As Quentin said, Adrian's mood depended a good deal on who he was with.

1935 was a momentous year for Adrian. By the beginning of the year it seems probable that he and Karin now occupied the same house – no. 50. This is confirmed by a visit from Ann in February, who came to dinner with the Woolfs, 'rather pale, rather resolute and melancholy perhaps'. She was going in for an exhibition at Newnham, and came to ask Virginia to vouch for her character. She hadn't even told her parents about it. 'Karin', Virginia wrote, 'only seen in bed in the morning, Adrian seldom, the house full of lodgers and patients.' A gloomy picture of family life; but it must be remembered that Ann tended to take a depressed view of it, and of life in general. Her cousin Barbara Strachey recalls that as a child her constant cry was, 'It isn't fair!'

Both parents were preoccupied with their own lives, except for holidays at the King's Head, to which parties of friends were happy to come, in spite of the primitive conditions and unappetising food. For the Blacketts and the Williams-Ellises, sailing was the chief attraction. Mrs Blackett did something to introduce more civilised ways of enjoying life there. A photograph shows her setting out tea for the children on the lawn. Giovanna Blackett, some years younger than the Stephen girls, visited the King's Head during the Twenties and Thirties and sensed what was to her a free, licentious atmosphere. Was there, she wonders now, 'much promiscuity?' She was conscious, as she put it, of Ann's and Judith's 'sexuality'. How, she wondered, did the uninhibited behaviour of the grown-ups strike the local, mostly agricultural people, the Bearders for instance who lived in a cottage opposite the King's Head? Whereas to Susan Henderson, brought up in her mother's world, life at the King's Head was as it was lived at home, in Gordon Square.

Giovanna's aunt, Marion Milner[67] (*née* Blackett) remembers more about Karin than Adrian. She recalls Karin driving her 'somewhat erratically' through Colchester, complaining that a colleague had suggested that she should not be allowed to give seminars, she was too irresponsible. 'Irresponsible!' she cried, waving her arms in the middle of the busy High Street.

Adrian's direct, uncompromising manner during the Society's meetings could give offence. Marion remembers coming away from one such meeting with Vera Meynell, then an analyst in training, who remarked, 'I don't like my friends being made fools of.'

Another friend was Gwenda David. As talent scout for the Viking Press she has given her life to the discovery and promotion of talented writers, one of the best-known and loved figures in the book trade. She became Karin's patient in 1934. She recalled an incident which shows the easy-going behaviour still possible even so late as in the 1930s between analyst and patient – though the Stephens were not typical members of their profession. Karin passed on to Adrian something she, Gwenda, had said during a session, and he repeated it at dinner with Virginia Woolf. When she and

[67] Sister of Lord (Sir Patrick) Blackett F.R.S., physicist, Nobel Prize winner 1948. Died 1974. The Blackett family sailed with Adrian and Karin.

Gwenda met Virginia said: 'I know all about you!' Karin agreed that it was a breach of confidence and apologised. Gwenda also remembers that once, during a session, Adrian came in with some chocolates and began throwing them to analyst and patient. 'He was eccentric, sometimes almost mad,' Gwenda thought.

Her analysis did not last long: after a week or two Karin said, 'This is ridiculous! Get off that couch and we can be friends!' Their friendship lasted till Karin's death. Gwenda, too, often visited the King's Head though it was still totally without any convenience. Once, when she was there with her children, they pointed to maggots crawling out of the cold meat. Karin insisted on eating it: 'Sailors used to – did them no harm!'

A patient of Karin's, Dr le Maré, spoke of Adrian and Karin as 'pioneers'. He spoke warmly of Karin, less so of Adrian. His sister, Adrian's patient, found him a 'cold fish'. She left him after six months. He himself went to Adrian, wanting to be taken on as a psychoanalytical candidate. All he can remember Adrian saying was: 'I can be objective.' (Unexplained.) He, too, found Adrian a cold fish. He reported Adrian as saying about a patient of his before the war, 'She chooses not to speak,' implying, Dr le Maré thought, that he, Adrian, 'could do nothing about that'. Karin, he said, was the guru or *éminence grise* of the Society of Creative Psychology, founded because psychoanalysis was 'in danger of taking away people's dignity'. The society collapsed on the outbreak of World War II.

Karin and Adrian were great joiners. They belonged, of course, to the British Psychological Society, also the British Society for the Study of Sex Psychology.[68] They were eclectic; they showed their resistance to Ernest Jones's orthodox limitations by their interest in the Tavistock Clinic,[69] which accepted Jungian practitioners as well as 'B Groupers' (Anna Freud's adherents) and Kleinians, and furthered the work of psychotherapists. Dr W. R. Bion was told he must leave the Tavistock if he wanted to remain in the Psychoanalytical Society. He continued to work at the Tavistock and kept his membership of the Society.

By the middle 1930s there are few references in Karin's letters to Mary Berenson about separation. The routine of their working day, alternating with sailing holidays at the King's Head, and Karin's occasional disappearances to Italy, or revisiting the United

[68] Dr Lesley A. Hall

[69] The Tavistock Clinic, founded in 1920 by Dr Hugh Crichton-Miller, was one of the first out-patient clinics to provide systematic major psychotherapy inspired by psychoanalytical therapy for out-patients unable to afford professional fees (*Fifty Years of The Tavistock Clinic*, H. V. Dicks).

States, and fleeting visits to Europe with unspecified friends – perhaps with J.F. – seemed to satisfy her need for freedom. Adrian tolerated her absences; he saw more of his Bloomsbury friends, and of his colleagues who liked him but were wary of Karin's forceful egocentricity.

As an active pacifist, Adrian was increasingly concerned about the situation in Europe, the rise of Mussolini and the Italian Fascists, the growing power of Hitler and the Nazis, and the weakness of the United Nations. When the League was founded in 1919 its purpose was to prevent war and promote collective security. But America never belonged, and the attempt to prevent war failed; sovereign States could not agree on joint action. When Italy invaded Abyssinia in 1935 sanctions were imposed on her, but with little effect. In the late 1930s, when the USSR became a member, their foreign minister, Litvinov, announced 'Peace is indivisible', which, for a time, put heart into the other members. The Hoare–Laval Pact, an empty gesture by the UK and France to halt the Italian war in Abyssinia, was ridiculed even by *The Times*, and the League seemed to be tailing away in empty gestures. In 1936 Leonard Woolf wrote to his nephew, Julian Bell: 'The League is dead. Collective security is rotten.' But Adrian, a member of the League of Nations Union, an organisation in Britain to support the League, stuck to his beliefs, and acted as best he could.

In 1934 a peace ballot was organised by the League of Nations Union and pacifist groups, and by Sir Stafford Cripps, a radical member of the Labour Party. 'The response was widespread throughout the country and produced an astonishing vote for disarmament, the abolition of the private manufacture and sale of arms, and the use of sanctions against an aggressor'.[70]

How Utopian that seemed then, how much more so today! But it was the kind of basic commonsense that appealed to Adrian's logical mind.

In October 1935 Virginia Woolf attended a peace conference 'by way of a joke'. It was not her scene, but very much her brother's. Adrian went with her to a party afterwards: 'A. very spruce and lively and witty. We hit it off when other people are there. I have the impression he is far more social than he was.'

In December 1935 Adrian held a meeting in 50 Gordon Square, with the idea of supporting French radicals by forming a British group, For Intellectual Liberty, a counterpart of an organisation of French antifascist intellectuals, *Le Comité de la Vigilance.*

[70] *The Life of Richard Stafford Cripps* by Colin Arthur Cooke, 1942.

In December 1936 he held another meeting to discuss, among other matters of international import, the situation in Spain, where the Republican government had been attacked by army rebels under General Franco. At a further meeting ways of helping the Spanish Republicans were discussed. With his medical background, working with Spanish Medical Aid, already established, would have been the appropriate medium. As analysts, he and Karin might have been prohibited from taking too public a part; but their friends and relatives became involved in support groups. A cousin, Janet Vaughan, a young doctor, certainly did. And Julian Bell's friend, Portia Holman, was a courier, travelling between London and Madrid. Soon Julian himself was to return from China to enlist as an ambulance driver.

The effect of the Spanish Civil War on people of all ages and classes was overwhelming, impossible to describe to anyone too young to have experienced it. Years later Dame Janet Vaughan, as she was by then, said in a television interview that the Spanish Civil War was the political event that had most affected her life.[71]

[71] *The Signal was Spain* by Jim Fyrth.

16

VIRGINIA'S DEATH

In March 1936, Adrian's 'queer' seizures began to recur. Twice Karin found him unconscious on the floor; when he came round he was violently sick. These episodes seem never to have been diagnosed; but it is probably that his heart was affected by the disease contracted so long ago while he was still at Cambridge.

'It is awful', Karin told Virginia, her usual confidante, 'finding him unconscious – awful when someone you are fond of is ill.'

'Yet she went away,' Virginia wrote in her diary. She herself would never have left someone she cared for who was ill. Her generosity of spirit was never more consistent than in her concern for her brother, perhaps with an admixture of guilt, at having neglected him when they were children, or perhaps for loving Thoby more, but wise, practical, marking Adrian's depression, his changes of mood, his sense of failure, rejoicing at his success; furthermore bearing with Karin; keeping an eye on them both.

In September 1937, Virginia wrote: 'Any news of A.? . . . Probably at Charleston recovering from an illness.' He had been in a nursing home, suffering from the heart trouble that had begun to plague him. As he wrote to Vanessa, 'my heart hammers in my chest'.

He and Karin had moved that year into 26 York Terrace, Regent's Park. And it was here that Marjorie Freeman, then married to John Freeman's son, Dick, came to know the Stephens; they often dined there. Marjorie took to Adrian, but didn't much care for Karin who asked Marjorie if she and Dick would take Adrian to the King's Head to recuperate after his illness. They were delighted at the idea, and with two other young friends set off for Essex.

Their weekend was most enjoyable, except for their qualms of uncertainty at Adrian's over-activity. They sailed; they played progressive ping-pong in the Long Room, a game demanding speed and a quick eye. To their alarm Adrian insisted on joining in! On Bank Holiday they went to the Fun Fair at Clacton. It was all new and delightful to Adrian, specially when Dick, a good shot, bagged a huge pink fluffy rabbit. And he relished Marjorie's cooking – not a usual feature of King's Head hospitality.

His recuperation was complete.[72]

Marjorie and Dick were among our many friends who threw all their energy into the Spanish cause. During these last pre-war years a curious dichotomy possessed our minds. On the one hand the German invasion of Great Britain seemed almost certain, with the likelihood of our death or at least subjection to all too-imaginable horrors so that one was in continual dread and fear, specially those of us with children. On the other hand everyone we knew shared a heady sense of liberation, of community, focusing our activity on supporting the Spanish struggle for survival, contributing such talent as we had, artists like Quentin Bell through the Artists International Association, musicians led by Alan Bush, Ralph Vaughan Williams, Adrian's distant cousin among them, voicing their support. Benjamin Britten and W. H. Auden collaborated on songs for a cabaret at a dance organised by the AIA.[73] Songs like 'I'm a jam tart' and 'Tell me the truth about love' were sung by Hedli Anderson, Louis MacNeice's wife. I cannot attempt to explain the split in our minds, only record it as I experienced it.

After General Franco's coup in an attempt to overthrow the newly established liberal government, and the outbreak of war in Spain in July 1936, Leonard Woolf supported the Republicans, and threw his energy into a vain attempt to influence the Labour Party: they remained uncommitted, following the non-interventionist policy of the British Government under Baldwin, who vetoed the supply of arms to Spain, and the dispatch of food ships.

The intervention of the German and Italian air forces on Franco's side added fresh impetus to the mobilisation of various forms of support. What caught people's imagination was the strategic bombing of civilians, the first time it had ever been tried in warfare. After the slaughter at Guernica, the British Government reluctantly allowed 4,000 Basque children to be shipped to Britain. On May 23, 1937, the first 2,000 landed at Southampton. Yvonne Kapp, Adrian's patient, was among the organisers of the camp from which

[72] Information from Marjorie Beadle.

[73] Artists International Association

they were dispersed to 'Basque Homes' hastily set up all over the country.[74] She also helped to organise the great Albert Hall meeting on June 24, 1937, under the auspices of the Joint Committee for Spanish Relief. There was widespread sympathy in Europe and the USA for the Republican cause, mostly among intellectuals and trade unionists, many of whom volunteered to go to Spain to help, either to fight or to drive ambulances and other such work. One of the earliest casualties was Julian Bell. He wrote from China that he intended to return and enlist in the International Brigade. Vanessa's consternation may be imagined. She always had a close relationship with her adored elder son.

Leonard Woolf wrote to Julian on February 19, 1937 that he had had an informal talk with the Spanish ambassador who told him that they did not want untrained volunteers. Anyone with skilled, technical knowledge was of immense value. Volunteers had come to him offering to drive lorries, but it was of no use if they did not speak Spanish.

Julian returned to Charleston and, as a compromise, volunteered as an ambulance driver (one of the most dangerous assignments). He left for Spain early in 1937. During the battle of Brunete, in July 1937, he and his companion were bombed from the air and took cover under their ambulance. But he was hit; shrapnel ripped off part of his rib-cage, exposing his lungs and heart. After a punishing ambulance journey over rough roads, two doctors, one of them Philip d'Arcy Hunt, a chest specialist, went to work on him. But he died in the night of July 18, reciting French poetry.

For Adrian, 1938 was an eventful year. In the summer Sigmund Freud and his daughter Anna, a child psychologist, came to London, and were joined by a number of analysts from Vienna and Berlin. Controversy soon arose between 'the B Group' and the supporters of Melanie Klein, who had the tactical advantage of having had ten or twelve years' establishment in the Society. Differences of approach to analysis, partly personal, partly professional, led to a schism that threatened the entire British Society. In a compromise worked out during and in spite of World War II, Adrian was to play a crucial rôle.

In the same year he was involved in an adventure that was very much to his inclination. Leonard Woolf describes it in a volume of his autobiography, *The Journey Not the Arrival Matters*:

> Just before the war Adrian Stephen learnt that a German

[74] Information by Yvonne Kapp

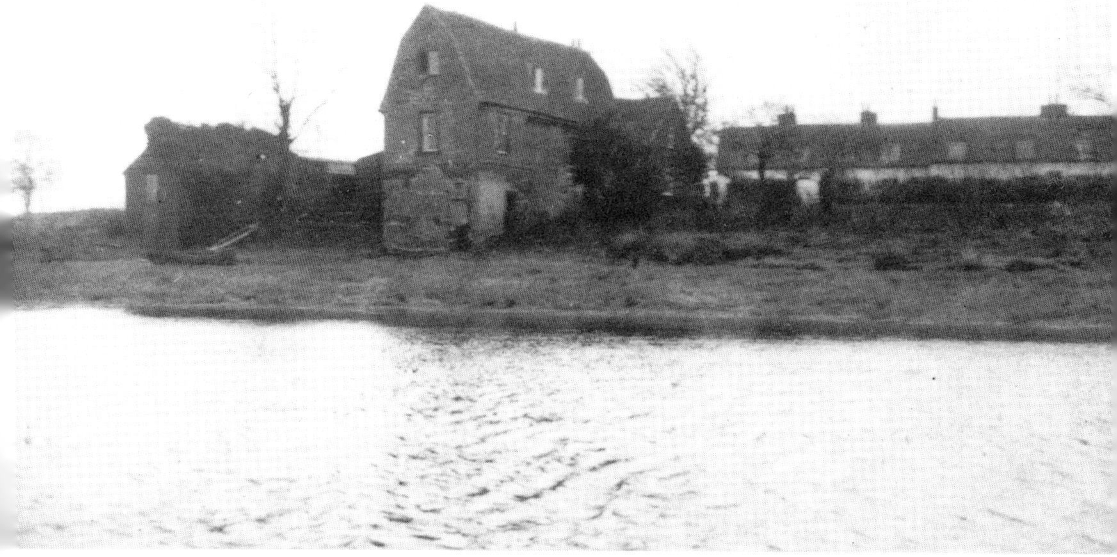

The King's Head was first rented then bought by Karin. The house stands on the shore of Hamford Water, the inland sea near Harwich on the Essex coast, on which Arthur Ransome's *Secret Water* is closely modelled. These photographs, like the others at this location, come from the Stephens' family album.

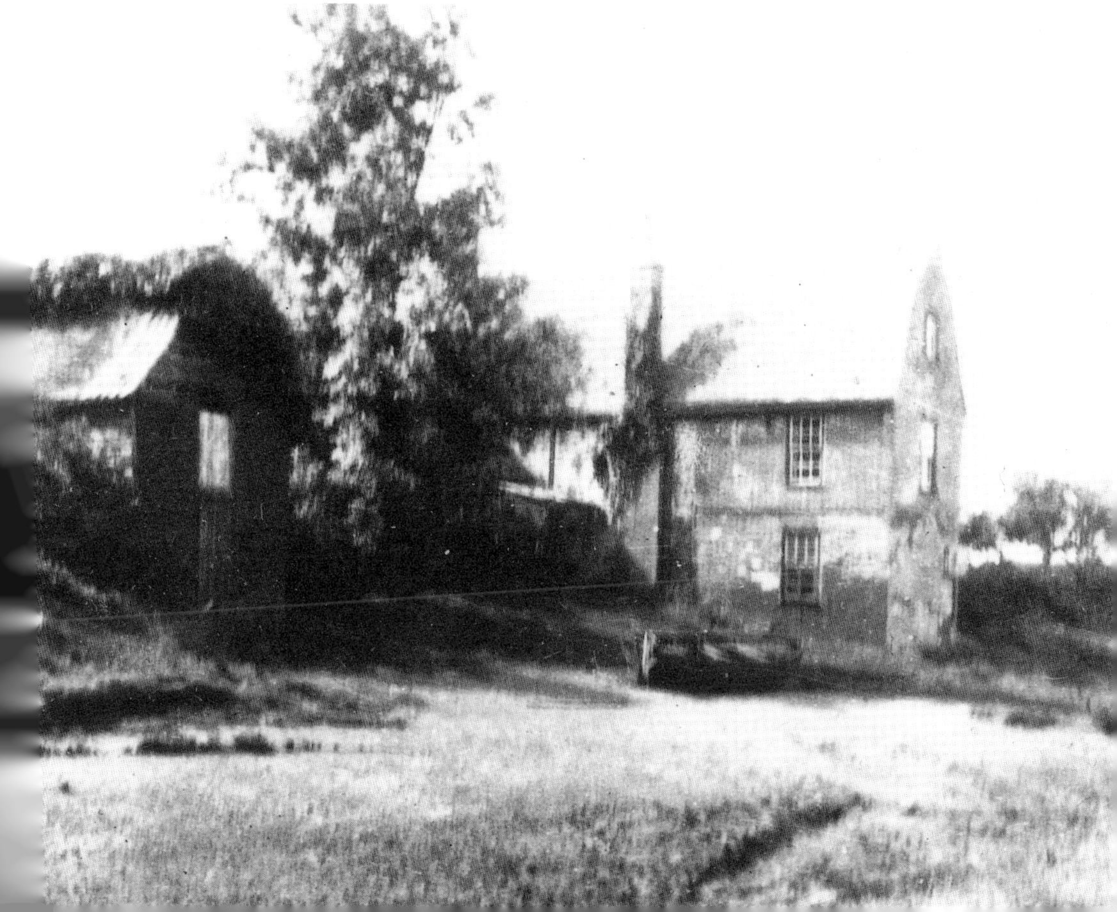

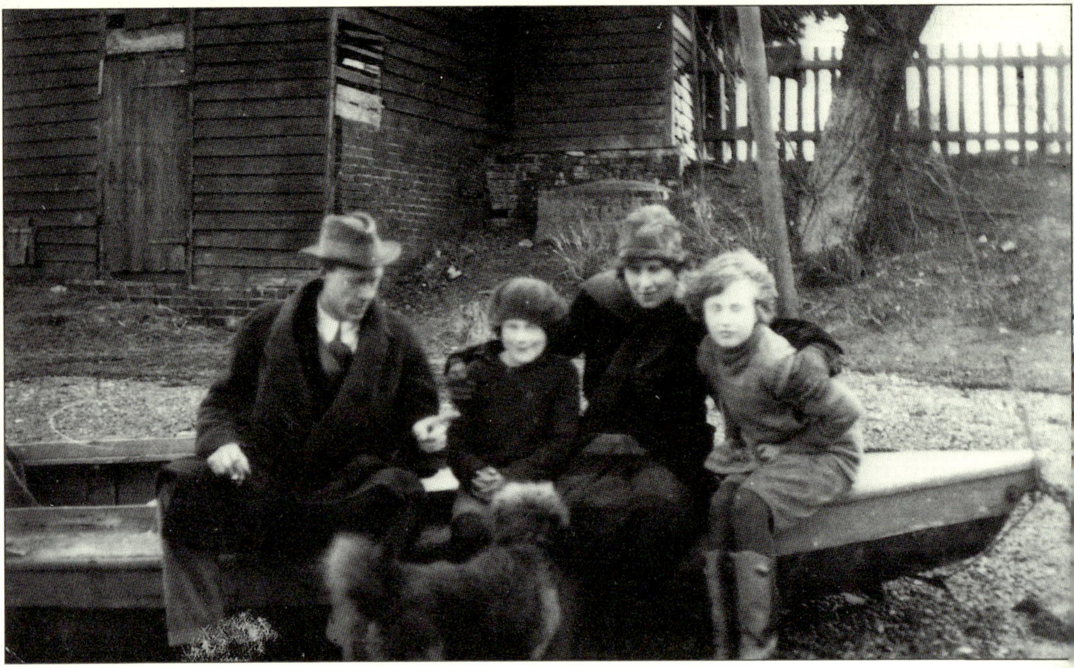

Left to right: Adrian, Judith, Karin and Ann at the King's Head. They are sitting on the dinghy left them by Logan Pearsall Smith – the *Shelduck*.

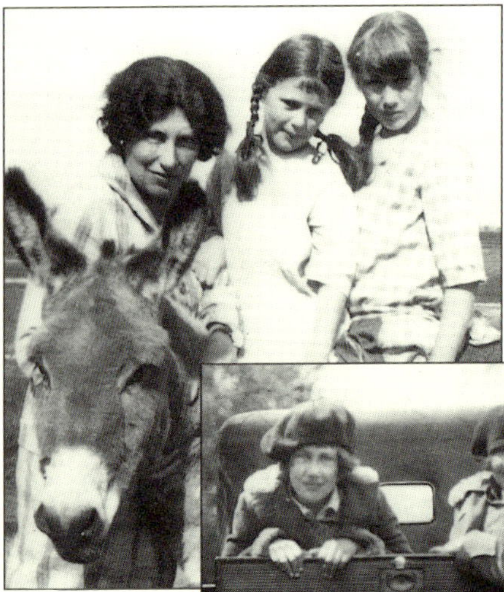

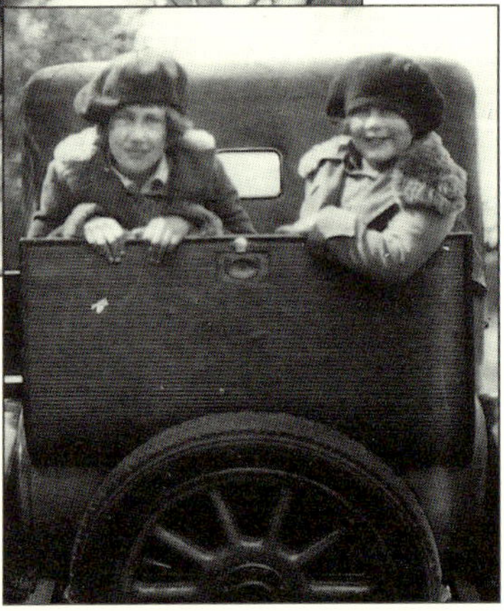

Above left: Karin with Ann and Judith.
Above right: Ann (left) and Judith

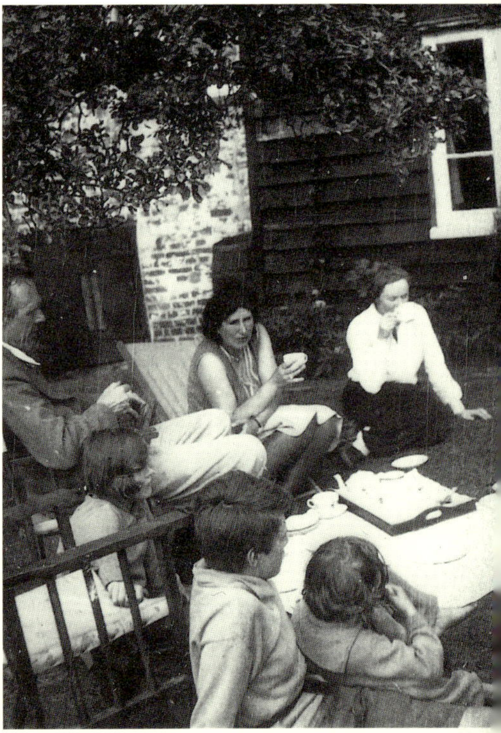

The first time at the King's Head. Adrian and Karin sit the boy and girl in the front are probably the Blackett children.

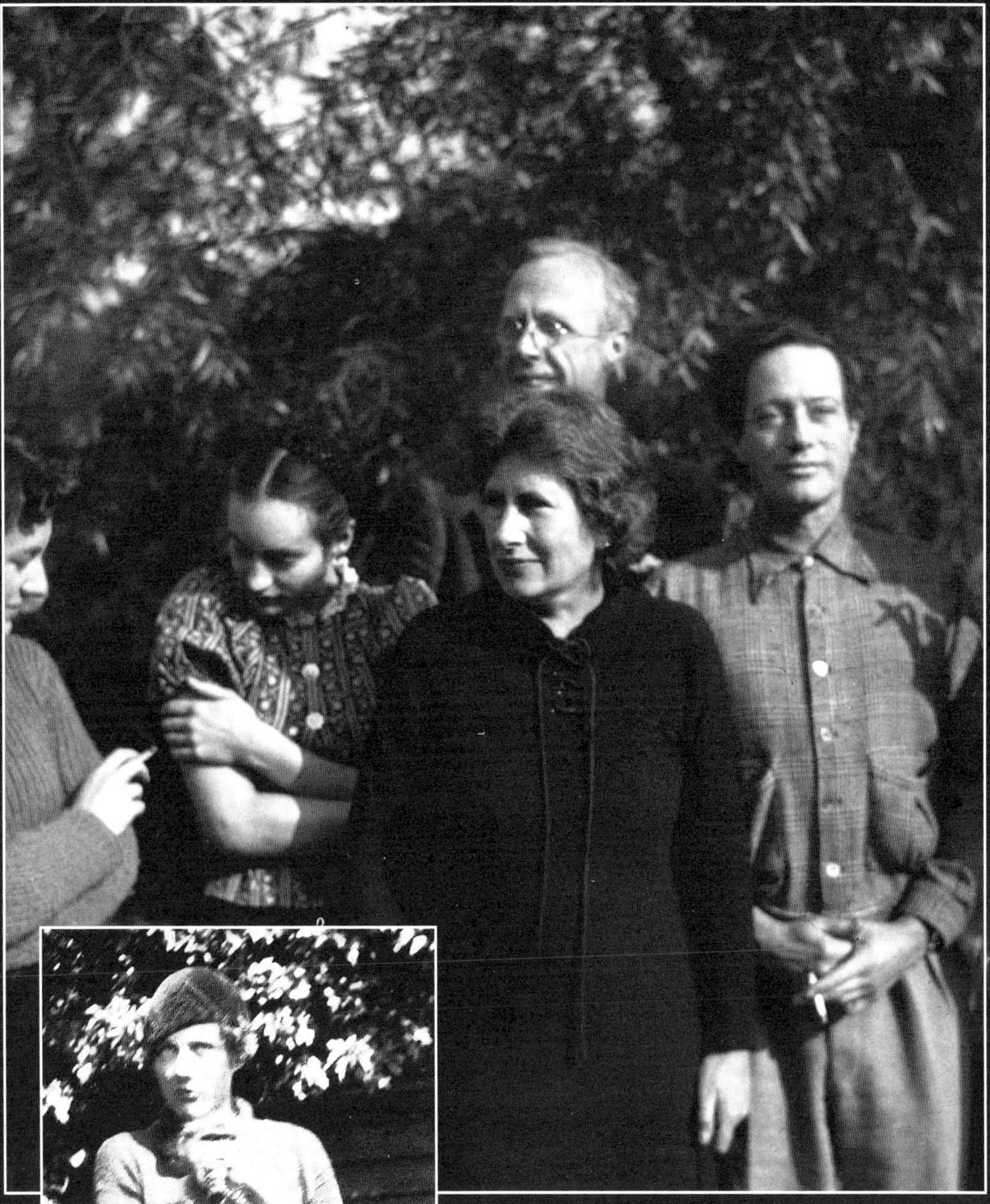

Duncan Grant with Adrian and Karin at the King's Head. The girl on Karin's right may be Judith.

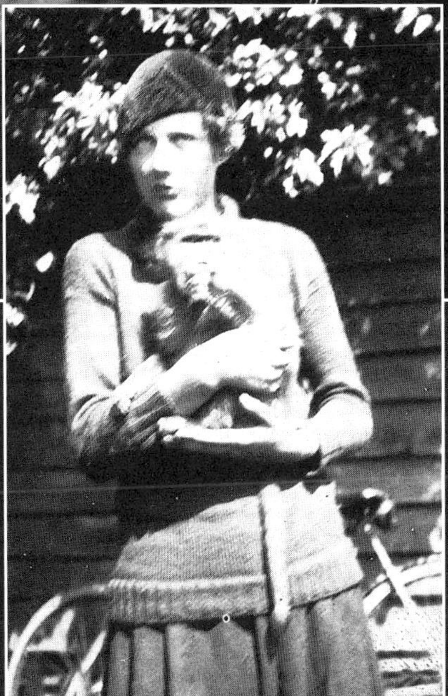

Ann with Sir Solly Zuckerman's baboon, which he brought with him to the King's Head. He was head of the London Zoo.

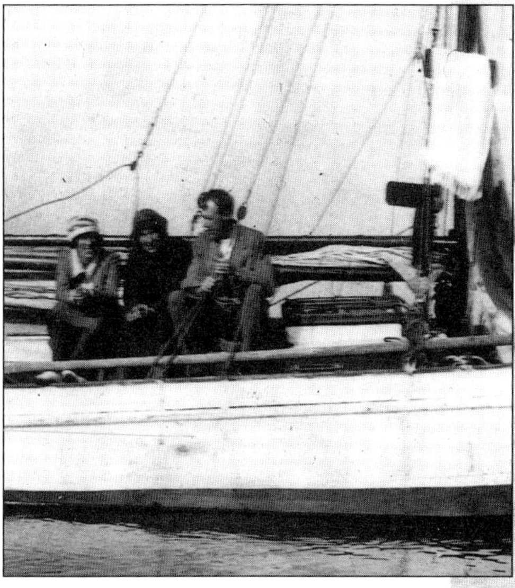

Adrian and Karin in the *Ran*, the boat they sailed across the North Sea and across the Thames Estuary. The figure on the left is unidentified. When he could not sleep at night Adrian would pick up in his imagination the light vessels, such as the *Kentish Knock*, they passed at night.

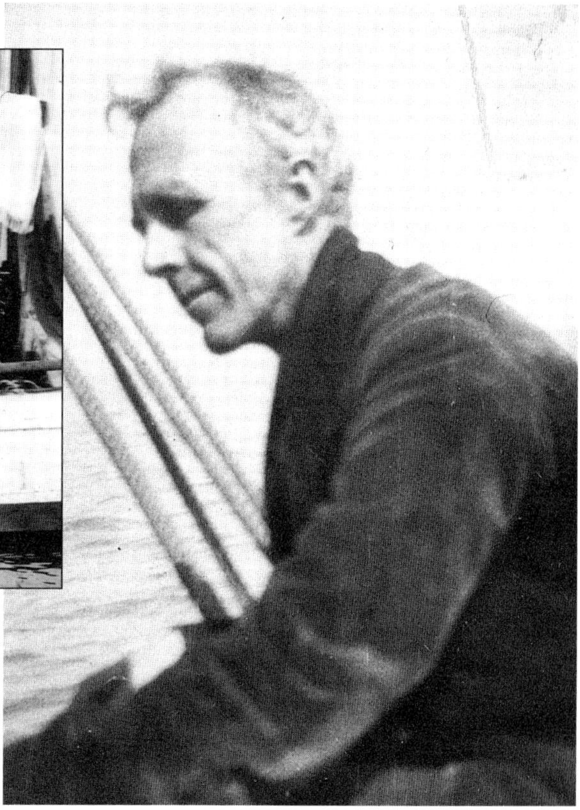

Above right Adrian sailing at the King's Head, 1937, having left a nursing home soon after heart trouble. As he wrote to Vanessa, 'My heart hammers in my chest.'

Below Adrian with Karin and Judith. It will have been noticed that he never wore traditional sailing clothes. He was always an unorthodox sailor.

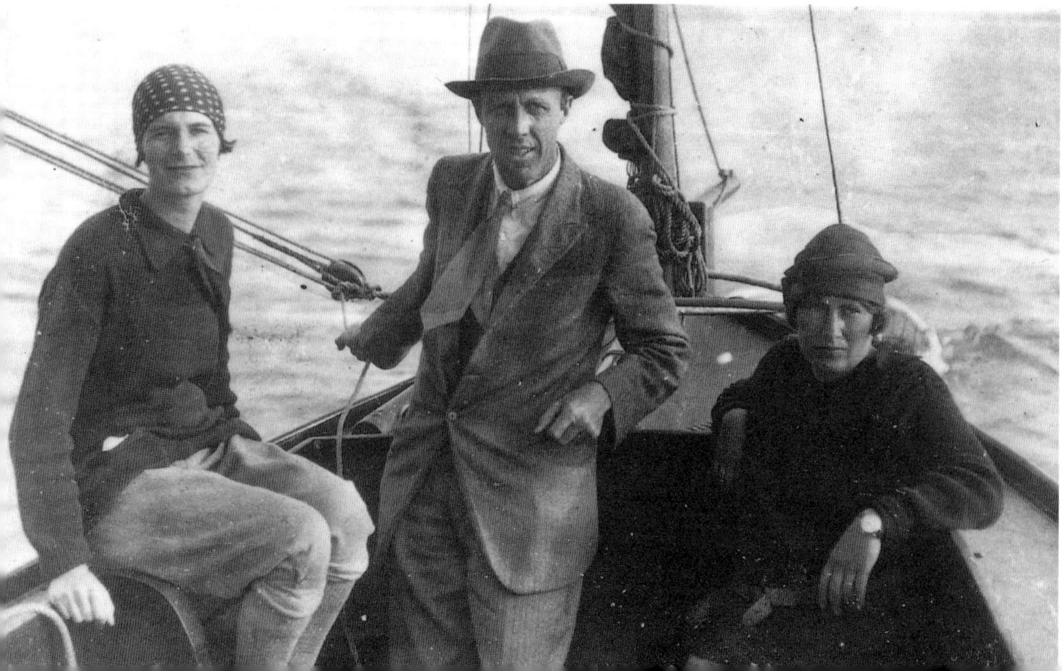

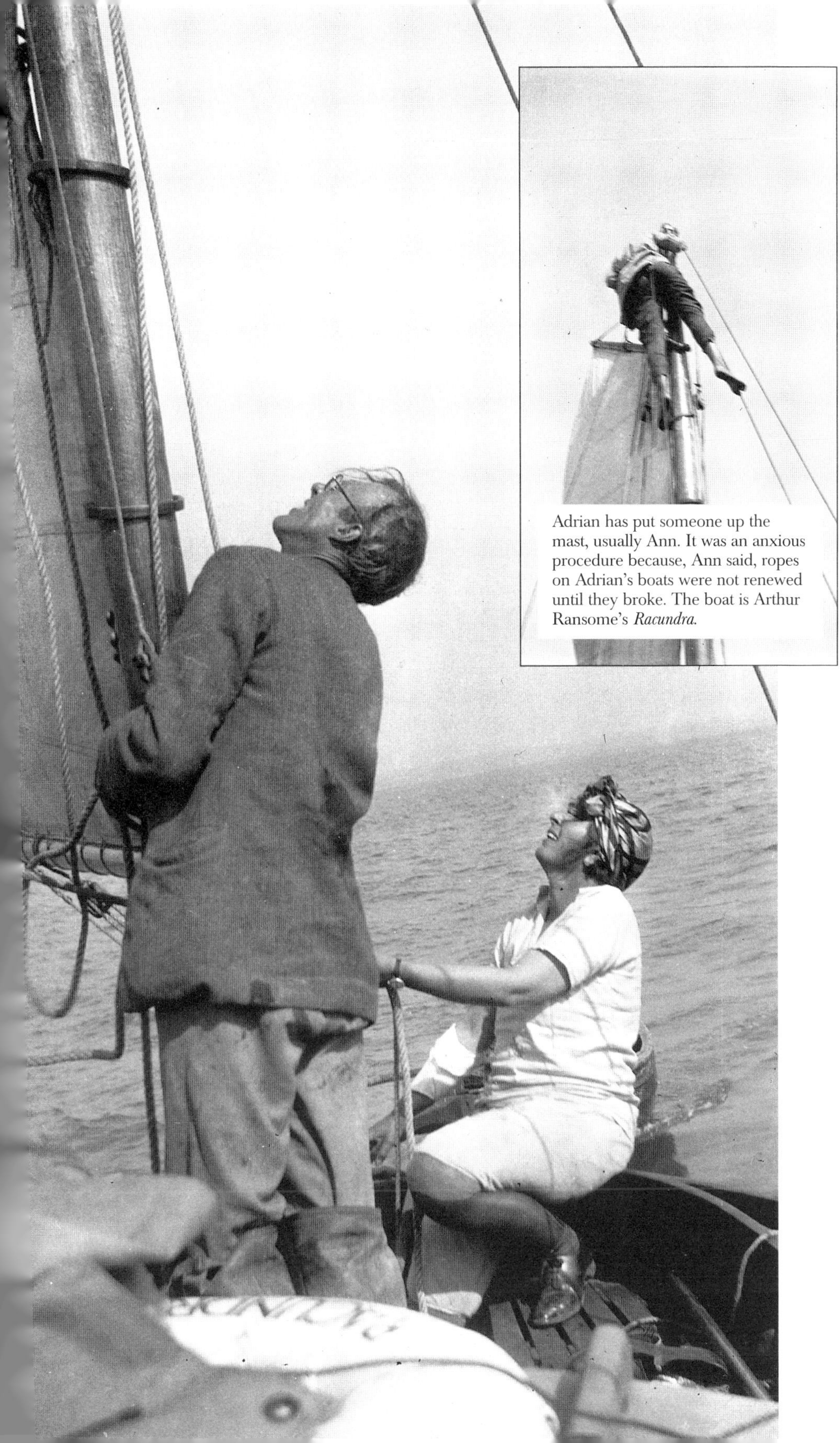

Adrian has put someone up the mast, usually Ann. It was an anxious procedure because, Ann said, ropes on Adrian's boats were not renewed until they broke. The boat is Arthur Ransome's *Racundra.*

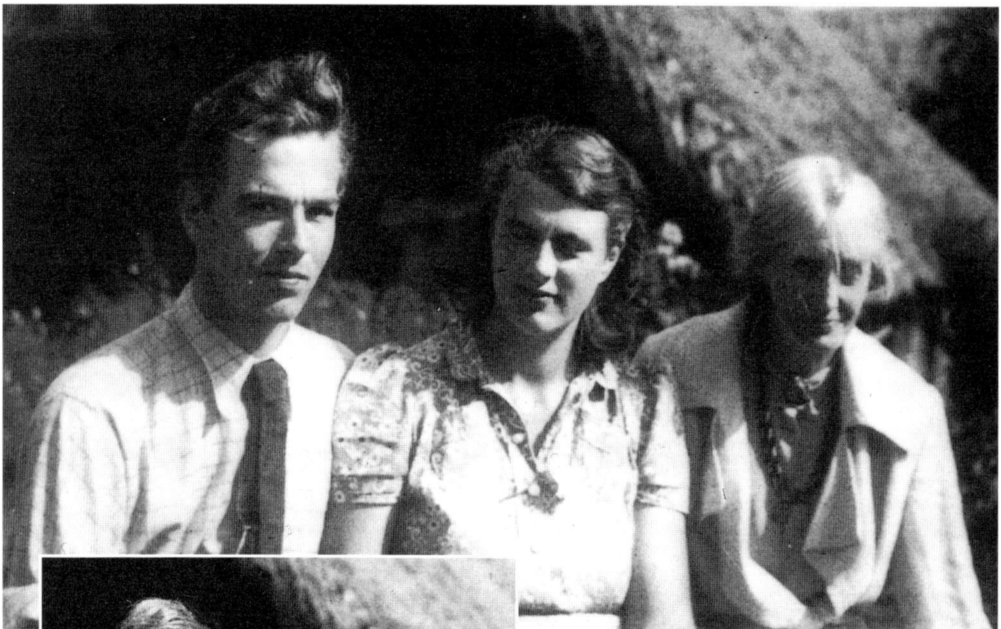

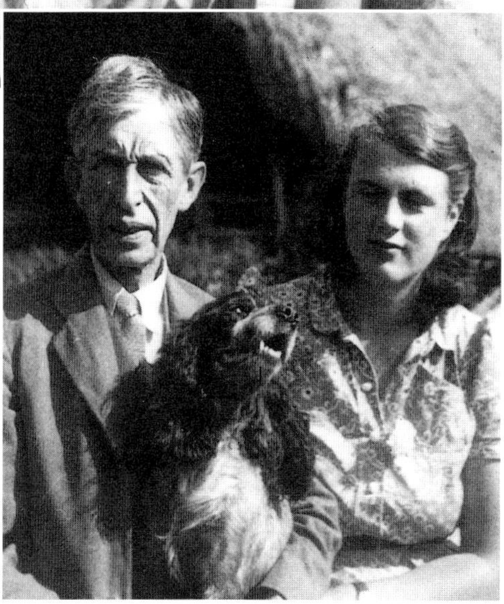

Judith with Virginia Woolf, and Judith's young man who died in the USA and . . .

with Leonard Woolf. Judith visited the Woolfs and the Bells but Ann felt she was 'not welcome'.

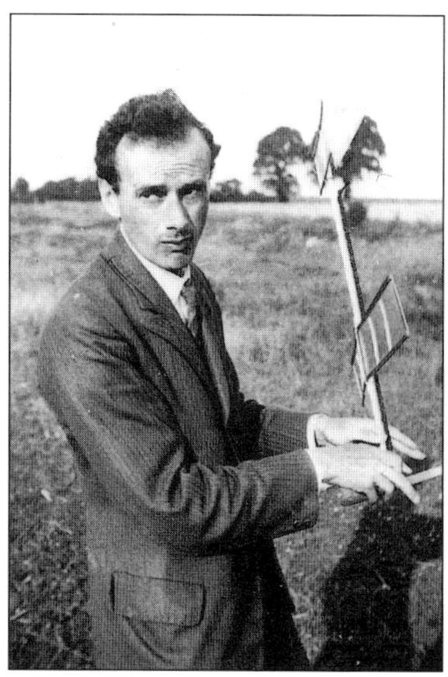

Patrick Blackett, the Nobel Prize-winning physicist. The Blackett family remember happy times there, sailing with Adrian, 'rather casually!'

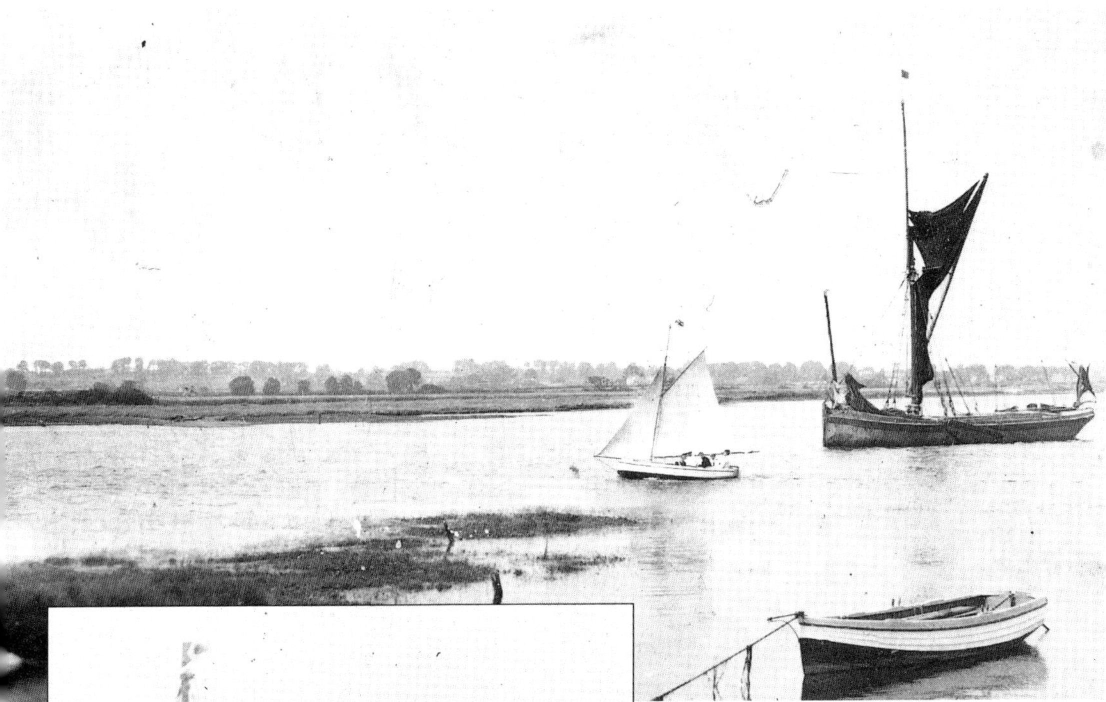

The view from the King's Head at high water. A Thames barge was an occasional but welcome visitor.

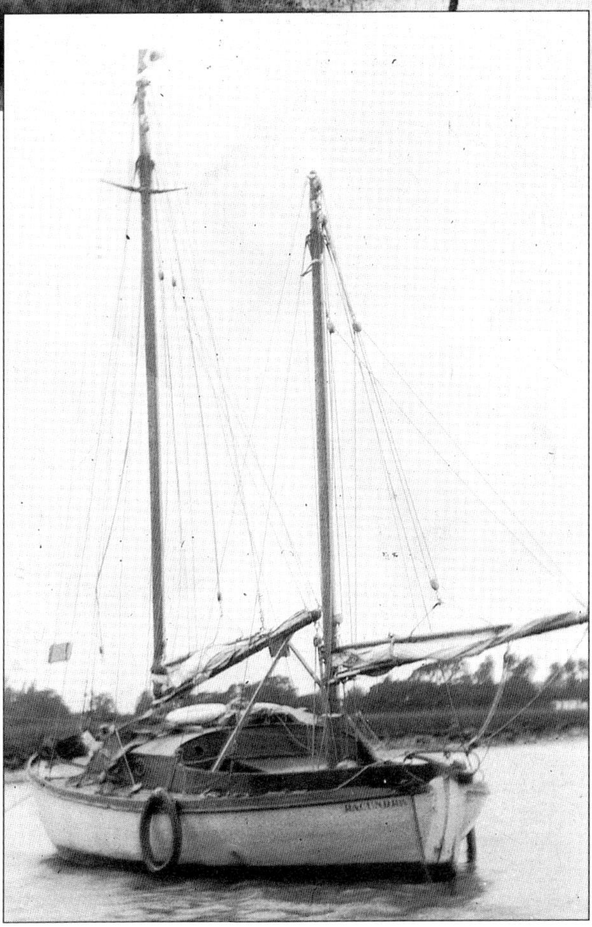

Arthur Ransome's *Racundra*, lent to Adrian and Karin, in Hamford Water.

Adrian and Skipper. Adrian never changed back into civilian clothes when off duty.

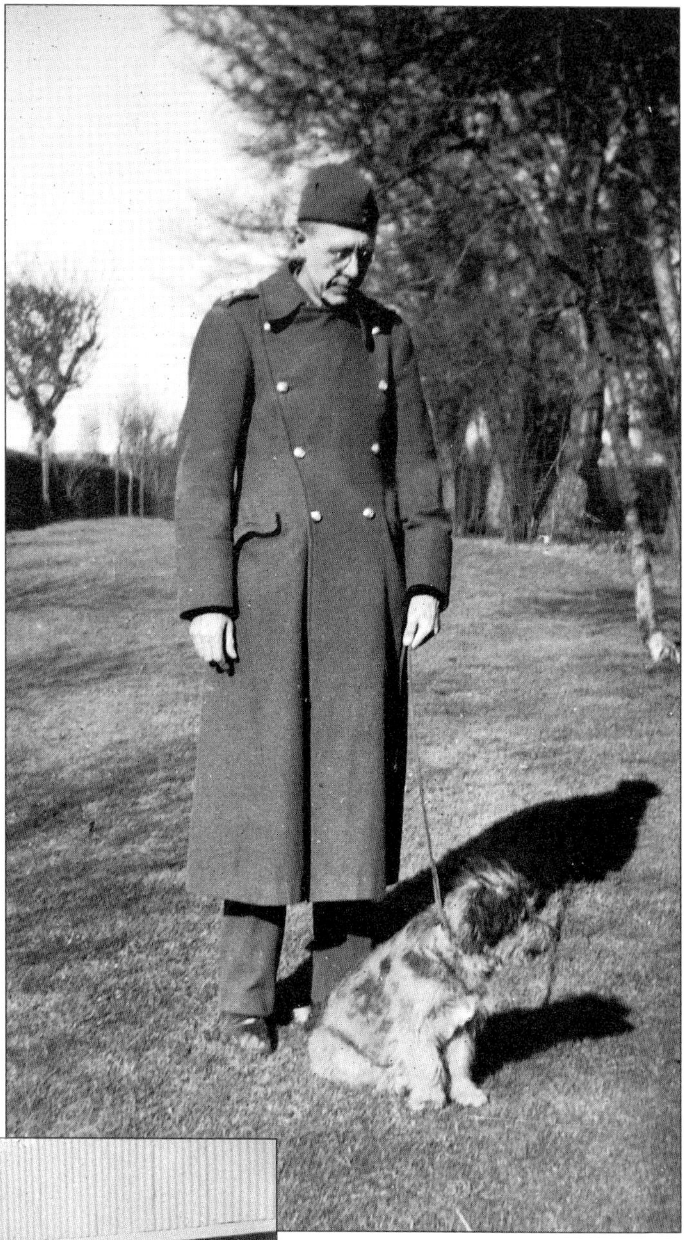

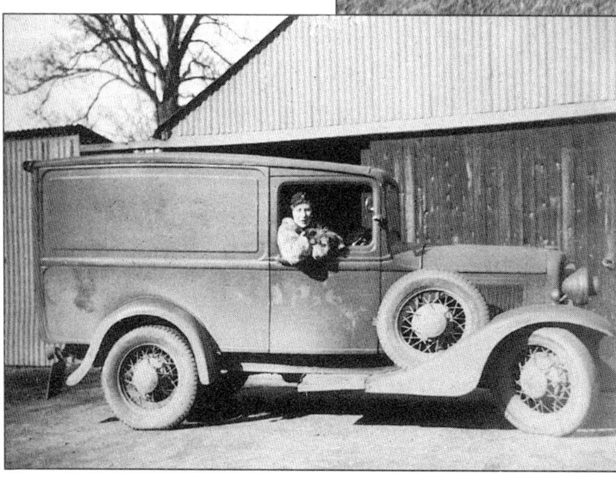

Karin in 'the old canteen van', 1941. She wrote to Leonard Woolf that she had arranged to do 'rather exciting' research at a Bristol mental hospital and for war work she had joined up as a driver in the Queen's Messengers Flying Squad Food Convoy, on call to go to any town in the West Country that had been badly blitzed.

> friend of his was in grave danger from the Nazis, and, with influential support behind him, he went to Berlin to try to get his friend out of Germany. He conducted some very strange and complicated negotiations in the course of which he saw something of what the Nazis were doing and meant to do, and also of the desperate plight of their victims. The account of his experiences still further opened one's eyes – one looked into the abyss.

The 'friend' was Carl von Ossietzky, a Nobel Peace Prize winner who had fought in World War I, an 'anti-militaristic Liberal' who edited the Berlin radical weekly *Die Weltbühne* and was well known for his opposition to the Nazi regime. He was urged to leave the country, but refused: 'Who wishes to fight the evil in his country must share that country's fate.' He was imprisoned after the Reichstag fire in 1933. An international campaign was mounted to 'free Ossietzky'.

Adrian's mission came to nothing. Ossietzky had been murdered in 1938.

But with his command of German Adrian visited Germany several times: it is more than likely that he was responsible for further negotiations on behalf of other refugees. His horror at what he saw of German brutality under Nazi rule so sickened him that he determined to have the means of suicide ready, in the all too likely event of war and a German invasion. Leonard Woolf writes that he also offered a prescription for the 'protective poison' to him and Virginia, who would certainly have been 'among the proscribed'. Harold Nicolson and Vita Sackville-West had taken similar precautions.

Then, came final defeat of Republican Spain, preceded by the shameful Munich Agreement on September 29, 1938, and followed by the invasion of Czechoslovakia in March 1939, putting an end to our fervid activities, but turning our attention to the bigger war that was coming, again, with a curious sense of relief mixed with dread.

Perhaps as a kind of farewell to the life they were leaving behind, Adrian and Karin gave a fancy-dress party in January 1939 at their Regent's Park house. Virginia went as Cleopatra.

She wrote in her diary:

> Adrian's party varied and no doubt successful. [Her list of guests is almost a roll-call of old and young friends.] Duncan

> a blond French princess. . . . Ann[75] almost naked, very distinguished lovely; aloof; fierce. [The Cecils,[76] David and Rachel were there.] And the usual bobbing corks on the waves – dullards hoping to get in touch with someone or thing & approaching & driven off & then attaching themselves: Portia Holman, the Enfields. A kind of liberation caused by wearing a mask, tipsiness and abandonment at not being one's usual self. . . . And we all on tiptoe, waiting Hitler's speech tonight.

She and Leonard attended the 25th anniversary dinner of the British Psychoanalytical Society on March 8 at the Savoy Hotel. At their table were Karin, Duncan Grant gossiping with Adrian, Vera Meynell, R. E. Money-Kyrle, psychoanalyst, one-time ace pilot in the Royal Flying Corps during World War I, who had just had a short book, *Superstition and Society*, published by the Hogarth Press; Rebecca West, and Mary Hutchinson, one-time companion of Clive Bell, were there; and Melanie Klein, also published by the Hogarth Press. Virginia describes her:

> A woman of character, & force & some submerged – how shall I say – not craft, but subtlety: something working underground. A pull, a twist, like an undertow: menacing. A bluff, grey-haired lady, with large, bright, imaginative eyes.

Adrian relinquished his pacifism. The coming war must be fought, Hitler overcome and his beloved Germany set free.

He volunteered to join the RAMC on November 26, 1939 – three months after the outbreak of war. But this did not prevent his engagement, throughout the conflict, in what has come to be called *The Freud–Klein Controversies, 1941–45*.[77] It had become apparent that the two factions in the Society, the supporters of Freud and his daughter Anna on the one hand, and on the other the adherents of Melanie Klein and her theories, had reached a pitch of animosity which threatened a split and so destroy the British Psychoanalytical Society. And it is a tribute to their civilised beliefs and their devotion to the psychoanalytic cause that the two groups, even as war

[75] Ann was married to Richard Llewelyn Davies on July 21, 1938. Adrian was not enthusiastic about his son-in-law. When war broke out, Ann, now a medical student, was doing her midwifery in Dublin where, at the time, her husband lived. He was one of the five sons adopted by J. M. Barrie, the writer and playwright.

[76] Lord David Cecil had just published *The Young Melbourne.*

[77] Pearl King and Riccardo Steiner.

broke out, agreed to meet and thrash out their rapidly becoming entrenched differences.

By the end of the Discussions in 1944, members of the Society had coagulated into three groups: the adherents of Anna Freud became known as 'B Group', those of Melanie Klein, 'Kleinians', and a third group, 'the Middle Group', composed of the analysts who did not want to take sides, to which Adrian and Karin belonged. The quarrels and the bitterness which appalled Adrian remained, though a compromise had been reached.

But that Karin, at least, sympathised with Melanie Klein and was against the attempt to exclude her from holding office is suggested by the following communication preserved in the archives of the Society and dated July 28, 1942:

> M KLEIN
> ADRIAN & I INTERESTED AGREE WITH YOUR LETTER. GLOVER BEHAVING LIKE A LUNATIC. PEOPLE ARE REALISING DANGEROUS FOR HIM TO STAY IN POWER. MADDENING FOR YOU GOOD IN LONG RUN. RE COMMITTEE ELECTION A & I TALKED WITH PAYNE & PRODUCED A LIST OF 5 WHO MIGHT SUPPORT YOU.
> MIGHT BE BEST NOT TO PRESS YOUR NAME EVEN THOUGH ANNA'S WAS PROPOSED. ABLE TO RELY ON FAIR DEAL & LESS OPPOSITION THAN IF PUT FORWARD BY YOURSELF. HOPE YOU AGREE.

Adrian made a major contribution to the controversial discussions. It is described in some detail in Appendix I.

Those were terrible years for Virginia. Every event, bringing the threat of war nearer, pressed upon her. From 1936 onwards her diary shows how fiercely she fought the threat of breakdown. As always, she sought sanity through work. She finished her biography of Roger Fry, reworked *Three Guineas*, and began her last novel, provisionally called *Pointz Hall*, then *Between the Acts*, published posthumously. Towards the end of her life, she regretted her lack of self-confidence, specifically in acquiescing in the decision that she should not bear children – a decision reached by consultants (and agreed by Leonard Woolf), though, surprisingly, not by her *bête noire*, Dr Savage.

Adrian was a psychiatrist, he had worked with psychotic patients at the Maudsley; he should have seen that she was referred to a psychiatrist trained to understand her condition and treat her, if necessary, with the drugs then available. His aloofness, his withdrawal, his failure to act as he ought are inexcusable.[78]

By the 1930s an analyst with a psychiatrist's training could at least have seen her every day, lightened the burden of her self-imposed attempt to be responsible for her own illness, her guilt at being ill, and the agonising sense of isolation, of being shut inside herself with her 'madness' (her word for her illness). He or she would have been there at the onset of a breakdown, and might have lessened its severity. For her 'madness' did not fall suddenly on her; her condition gradually worsened, as she was well aware, though she persistently denied it, perhaps partly because she dreaded the inevitable 'treatment'.

On March 28, 1941, knowing she was entering into another bout of illness from which she felt she would never recover and would continue to 'spoil his life', she walked down to the River Ouse, weighted her pocket with a large stone and drowned herself.

There is no record of Adrian's immediate response to her courageous well-considered death. At the time he was at the King's Head awaiting his call-up. But in April, 1941 he wrote to Vanessa:

> I had actually seen in some Sunday paper about Virginia's body, but thank you for telling me. You must have been having an absolutely ghastly time; and I wish I could do anything about it but I don't see what use I can be. In a way, of course, the whole thing is very unreal to me as I have been so far away from it all & living such an unnatural life as an officer of sorts. It is like a distant dream. For a good many years I had not heard . . . much of her and of course had never been nearly as close to her as you have always been so that anyhow it could not effect me like you. Since about 1914 in fact I have seen her rather seldom and have never been quite sure that she wanted to see me when we did meet. On the other hand in many ways the life before 1914 seems more real than the life since then. Hyde Park Gate and St Ives are extraordinarily vivid and so are the days which, I suppose, ought to be called 'Early Bloomsbury'. It does seem odd that, as you say, we are the only people left to remember our childhood. One great change is, I suppose, that one has become so much more of a spectator – at any rate I have. It is not that I feel an outsider myself but almost everyone else seems to be outside any life that is worth living. I suppose

[78] Dr Leslie Sohn in conversation.

> you still see a good many people who live reasonable lives but I find I cannot take people like army officers or most doctors seriously. They are some of them very nice, I suppose, but they are more like machines & less like human beings than most of the beasts in the zoo. I feel outside their life as one feels outside the lives of crocodiles – hippopotamuses. If they come too near one says a kind word or two & steps on one side to let them pass by. The Colonel here is exactly like a rhinoceros & behaves in the most unbelievable ways, it is a perpetual surprise to find out that he has been trained to speak.
>
> I wish that you and Duncan or either of you would come here for a bit. We have taken this house. It is in a very quiet sleepy village and you could do as much painting or whatever else you liked and it would be a change which I am sure you must need. Do try & come – we have got our own cook & would make you quite comfortable & you need not see anything of anyone you did not want to see. Love from Adrian.

He wrote again in May:

> I have been thinking about the inhabitants of 'Old Bloomsbury'. I suppose that as far as we were concerned it began, as you say, when we emigrated there in 1904 but I suppose there must have been something there when we got there. There was already, I suppose, a colony in the Fitzroy St. region which more or less centred round the Slade – but perhaps that did not actually form part of what later became 'Bloomsbury' though, of course, Roger was hanging about somewhere. I don't think he can really have come into 'Bloomsbury', therefore, before about 1908 or 9.

17

WARTIME

Adrian wrote to Vanessa on June 24, 1940 that he and Karin were still going on with 'the remnants of their practices' but they would cease when air-raids began seriously. 'We are also air raid wardens . . . and sit on two evenings a week in a basement with a curious collection of individuals, an ex-submarine commander, an estate agent, a chauffeur, two or three women clerks.' If a raid begins they have to 'stand by' and they have to go out to rescue people from fires and direct the traffic and 'take control generally of any "incident". It is quite amusing work really because one meets such queer people.'

They also had the job of dealing with psychological 'casualties' at a first-aid post at the Middlesex Hospital. The advantage of that work was that they would be paid for it. 'I can imagine the inhabitants of Charlotte Street becoming very excited. Our official instructions are to treat them with firmness, to appeal to their patriotism (they will very likely be Italians) and to give them Bromide and Morphia and send them home as soon as possible.'

On August 26, 1940, he was given an emergency commission as a lieutenant in the Royal Army Medical Corps (RAMC). Adrian, who so hated militarism, whose contempt as a young man had been expressed in elaborate and ingenious hoaxes, poking fun at authority, was now a number, P/146426, in a vast authoritarian organisation, fitted out in khaki battledress which could not be made to fit – for a time he wore his own flannels – 'posted to 1st Depot for Course of Instruction'. If this included the drill, square-bashing and shouting of orders which so nonplussed his friend Julian Trevelyan, the painter, that he had a whole platoon in dire confusion, how would Adrian have fared?

He didn't generally find his fellow officers congenial. He wrote to Vanessa from his WOSB office on August 28, 1944:

> It is very difficult not to be anti-Semitic when one meets people. As a matter of fact I think the real thing that saves me is the absurd and violent anti-Semitism of some of the officers I meet. I often find myself asking them why on earth they are fighting on the English side in this war. They are like a lot of idiotic schoolboys of 14 or of savages who are terrified of neighbouring tribes & cannot understand that their own is not necessarily the best in all ways. It is quite extraordinary, they all say that they want to wipe out the 'Huns' & that they want the whole country in ruins & on the other hand Germany is the one country they want us to copy – everyone else but a German is an inferior 'Wop' or 'Dago' or something.

In a fortnight he got his first posting to a military hospital in Glasgow. He took against the Scots from the first. (When I, proud of my native country, remarked 'But they're so friendly,' he retorted, 'That's what's so beastly.') He had his fill of that alien country, being shuttled between Glasgow and Edinburgh, to one psychiatric department after another, sometimes for not more than three or four days, for the army, like the entire country, had been thrown into readiness for battle. Confusion was inevitable. He was posted as Assistant Medical Officer in the Glasgow area on September 4, nine days later to a military hospital. Finally he landed up in the military hospital in Larbert, Stirlingshire, on December 14 till, on January 9, 1941, he was admitted to the Base Hospital suffering from pneumonia, which nearly killed him. (His daughter, Ann, remembered his being too tall for his military bed, so that his feet stuck out on a chair.)

From Kildonan Castle, Barrhill, near Girvan, Ayrshire, he wrote to Vanessa on February 19, 1941:

> A few days ago I was sent to this extraordinary place which has been turned into a convalescent home for officers. It is a large Tudor mansion . . . built by a millionaire . . . rather like a seaside hotel, it has a private golf course . . . and arrangements for every sort of game you can imagine . . . only about 8 other convalescents . . . taken individually . . . quite pleasant people, taken en masse they are just that collection of

> middle-class snobs which exactly suits the surroundings. I hope to be allowed out in a week or two and given some sick leave to complete my recovery in England. . . . It was a very queer experience being as ill as I was & to realise that the doctors were rather expecting me to pop off. I was apparently pretty delirious for a time which I can only vaguely remember and then there was a real death-bed scene with Karin & two or three doctors & some nurses standing round my bed while I had oxygen pumped into me and brandy poured down my throat . . . I did not think I probably should die that night. Poor Karin had rather a bad time of it, I am afraid, especially when the specialist told her one day that the whole thing would be settled one way or another within the next 12 hours. He turned out to be quite right as my temperature came tumbling down and I have been getting steadily better ever since.

After a spell at Kildonan his remarkably rapid recovery allowed him to return to military duties and he was posted to an RAMC training establishment, Boyce Barracks, Aldershot. From there, in April, he went to no. 41 General Hospital, Sandhill Park, Bishop's Lydeard, near Taunton, Somerset

On September 4 Karin wrote to Leonard Woolf from Court House, Ash Priors, near Taunton. They had had the luck to get a very charming house with a nice garden, only six or seven minutes' walk across the fields from Adrian's hospital. 'It is a pity the army are so full of red tape. Adrian's job ought to be first-class, but it seems there are so many distractions that he hardly ever gets a chance to do any work with the patients!'

Karin had hoped to 'work in with Adrian's hospital'; failing this she had arranged to do a 'rather exciting piece of research work at a large mental hospital near Bristol. For war work I have joined up as a driver in the Queen's Messengers Flying Squad Food Convoy. We have 8 milk-white lorries camouflaged in sky blue and are on call to go to any town in the West Country which may get badly blitzed. . . . All is quiet for the moment but I have little doubt that we shall get plenty of work bye and bye.' (Bristol was badly bombed in 1941; and Plymouth was laid flat, so that even people who knew the place could not find their way about.) She thanks Leonard for inviting Judith, who worked in London, down for weekends. 'I am afraid London may be badly blitzed again this autumn or winter . . .

your invitation will be a great blessing to her.' She ends: 'I did not write to you at the time about Virginia's death because I thought you wouldn't like to be troubled with letters which are of little help, but you know you had my sympathy.'

He and Karin had a pleasant enough life at Ash Priors. During his absence in Scotland she had worked in a civilian mental hospital in Shenley, Herts. He had missed her and family life, he said. Also they had congenial company. Emanuel Miller, the eminent psychiatrist (by now Lt.-Col. Miller), was working at a hospital at Norton Fitzwarren, and bicycled there from Bishop's Lydeard, where he lived with Betty Miller, already a distinguished writer, and their children Jonathan and Sarah.

In 1959 Betty wrote to Sir John Verney, sending him a copy of her novel, *On the Side of the Angels*, just published:

> By the way, Major McRae who appears now and then in the book is based on Adrian Stephen – Virginia's brother, he was an immensely tall man, & the army couldn't find a uniform big enough for him. He was a most civilised & witty person – & he and I got on very well together. He had a delightful slow wit – & when telling a story would open wide his blue astonished-looking eyes with the most comical effect. One evening at the officers club a lot of Polish officers came in. I said to Adrian 'I wonder what they think of Taunton?' The blue eyes opened even wider – 'Oo-h – I don't know,' he said at last – 'it may be that Taunton is more like Poland than we think.'

As 'Major McRae' resembles Adrian closely, these extracts from Betty Miller's novel are relevant, so well observed are her impressions of Adrian:

> A tall etiolated man, he was protected from animosity and ardour alike by that innate indifference to human affairs which he owed, in no small measure, to the peculiarities of his own physique. Oddly enough, this indifference which he never attempted to conceal, far from alienating others, attracted towards him their interest and goodwill: he was universally popular in the hospital where everyone from the C.O. downwards confided in old Mac, who took no sides and repeated no gossip. 'I must do some work, I suppose.

> You know how it is. The combined urine of the Western Command awaits my inspection.' And off he went down the gloomy corridor with the floating, inconsequent gait of a man who is not altogether aware of, less constricted in any way, by the limitations or peculiarities of his surroundings.
> 'I sometimes think', said Major McRae to Matron – he danced or rather he walked, he ambled along, as if instead of leading he were apologetically retreating from the partner whose co-operation he had sought – 'that the whole human race is a little mad.'[79]

And it was in 1942 that my husband, James, attached to VIII Corps HQ near Taunton, and I were introduced by Julian Trevelyan to the Stephens.

Then he and Karin moved away, on May 11, 1942, to Birmingham as the Bishop's Lydeard hospital was scheduled to move there. But the plan was cancelled and on May 15 he was posted to the military hospital at Shenley in Hertfordshire, as a 'specialist psychiatrist'. Karin could resume her work at the Shenley civilian mental hospital, and they found friends, including the Millers who were billeted at Garston, near Watford.

On 13 June, he had written to Vanessa about their move from Birmingham to Shenley. 'I have been moved again. I rather think it may have been in consequence of a letter I wrote to the War Office . . . criticising the plans for the new hospital at Birmingham. I got a quite polite letter back but it ended . . . that I should be moved somewhere else.' He must have been awkward to deal with: in the army, specially in 1942 when invasion seemed imminent, soldiers obeyed orders. The basic trouble seems to have been that he hated Birmingham. (Had he stayed he might have done interesting work with his colleague and friend, John Rickman who, with W. R. Bion, from the Tavistock Clinic, set up the first therapeutic community in a hospital.)[80]

He had been frequently in London, he writes, 'to fight battles for the Psychoanalytical Society. I believe I have won the first round against the opposition of the President and most of the committee to vote in favour of a committee to review our rules and make it compulsory for officers to retire from office periodically. I am afraid all that does not interest you but I find that in my old age I have become quite a good fighter. That miserable James Strachey, lick-

[79] *On the Side of the Angels* by Betty Miller (Robert Hale, 1945; Virago 1985).
[80] *British Psychoanalysts during the Second World War* by Pearl King.

spittle that he is, was against me – I think because his practice depends on the goodwill of Jones and Glover, as were some of the others in the same plight but unless the voting from absent members by post turns very heavily the opposite way to the rest of the voting my side has won. It is odd how pleased I feel, but I have had this row brewing for years and have always been persuaded against really starting it because the time was not right.'

(This refers to an event (dealt with in Appendix I) which was so crucial to him, and to the Society.)

The fact that he, a man of nearly sixty, in poor health, managed to combine army service with taking part in the Society's vital discussions throughout the war is evidence of his persistence, his capacity for unremitting activity reminiscent of his father. A less attractive characteristic, also shared with his father, was his habit of complaining. His family thought it derived from his mother's overindulgence.

In August, 1942 he was posted to Edinburgh, to No. 1 War Office Selection Board, where he examined candidates to assess their fitness to become officers, more satisfying and useful than treating, too late to be effective, casualties who did not want to be treated. This posting had been at his own request. Yet even here he found grounds for complaint – he had asked to be posted to London! But he was consoled by meeting an old family friend, Dick Rendel and his wife Judy. Dick was a Strachey on his mother's side. Elinor Strachey was the eldest of the family who lived at 51 Gordon Square, next door to the Stephens. Lt.-Col. Richard Rendel, like his grandfather, was a regular soldier, retired but recalled to take charge of Dover Castle in 1940 at the time of the retreat from Dunkirk. His detachment was shockingly ill-equipped. They had one anti-aircraft gun which he had asked for 'to keep up the morale of his troops'. He had been posted to Edinburgh at the suggestion of Lt.-Col. T. G. F. Rogers, consultant psychiatrist to the army, to advise on the value of the assessment of 'officer material' using psychological methods. (Germany had used advanced methods in officer selection since 1926.) Various experimental 'Wosbies' as they were instantly named, had been tried in different parts of the country. The Experimental Board formed in January, 1942 became No. 1 WOSB under the command of the psychologist, Lt.-Col. J. R. Sutherland.[81]

Through the Rendels Adrian met congenial friends, and his time in Edinburgh was not without compensations, though he still

[81] *Psychiatry in the British Army in the Second World War* by R. H. Ahrenfeldt.

hankered after a return to London. But he enjoyed the work. 'It isn't difficult', he wrote to me, 'picking out men who can be relied on to last out, and those who will be useful for a bit, then crack up.'

His letters to Vanessa include family matters specially when he was far from 'home' – i.e. London – and missing such rudimentary family life as he and Karin between them were able to provide.

In September 1941 he had written from Taunton: 'To our immense relief Ann has at last left Richard [her first husband]. . . . At the moment she is living with another young man who is a scientist of some sort and said to be very good at his job. . . . I quite liked him, though, if he is a diamond at all, he is certainly a rough diamond. He has a queer nervous grin which puts one off terribly at first and seems a little naively enthusiastic about Communism like most people of that particular age (he is 25) but he is certainly a great improvement on Richard.'

The scientist was Dick Synge, a brilliant chemist who, with his fellow scientist, Archer Martin, invented the technique of partition chromotography which revolutionised analytical chemistry. For this they were awarded a Nobel Prize in 1952. He and Ann married and had eight children. Judith and her husband Nigel Henderson had four. Adrian did not live to see them all. But I think he would have been gratified, given his feeling for families and family life, to have grandsired such a prolific continuation of the Stephen dynasty, albeit through the female line.

In another letter to Vanessa from Edinburgh on November 29, 1942, family matters crop up again:

> I was in London last week and saw Angelica at Judith's party. She was very charming and looking very beautiful, and I could not help feeling that Bunny was, as people used to say, 'unworthy of her'. But I suppose it is all right if she is happy. Bunny himself seemed a bit ossified.
>
> I wonder if you have heard about my daughters – Ann is expecting an illegitimate baby by her new young man and Judith has jilted Les and engaged herself to Nigel Henderson. Nigel is certainly an improvement on Les – but I think he is rather a feeble character, though they say he is much improved in the last year or two while he has been in the Air Force. I find it very hard to congratulate her but I suppose I shall have to.

At the end of February, 1943, he was posted to the Home Psychiatric Pool, London. As he wrote to Vanessa, parochial Londoner that he was, he had at last returned to 'civilisation'. This enabled him and Karin to remove all their removables once more – they never took unfurnished accommodation, however brief their sojourn – to the top floor of 59 Gordon Square, attended by the faithful Lottie whom Karin had once turned out so that she had had to take refuge with the Woolfs.

Adrian writes in high good humour to Vanessa on August 6, 1944:

> I don't know whether you will remember the battles I was waging in the Psycho-Analytical Society when I was last at Charleston – any how I am glad to say that they have ended in a complete victory – Jones who was President has resigned, he would very probably have any how on account of old age but Glover who was 'Scientific Secretary' has also resigned. It has all been great fun – I have never fought a battle like that in my life before and I never dreamt it would be so successful – Since he was driven out Glover has been blackguarding what he calls 'Army Psychiatrists' which means me more than anyone in every newspaper from *Horizon* to the *Daily Mail* and *Calvacade.*
>
> It looks as if this war would be over soon – I can't believe the Germans will hold out more than 2 or 3 weeks. Patrick Blackett, one of the chief scientific advisers to the Admiralty & War Office said about a fortnight ago said that he thought the most likely time was in 2½ months from then and he is not usually over sanguine. I think too much of our life.

On August 24, 1944, he writes to Vanessa from No. 20 WOSB, 39 Frognal, that he has an interim job, 'pleasant for a change', which shows the consideration shown by the army to personnel, even though the war was still being bitterly fought across Europe after the landings on D-Day.

'I have to interview officers who for some reason or other are out of a job and to give an opinion as to whether they are employable any more and what for.'

He goes on to say that he has 'wangled' a new job choosing people to demobilise the German Army and to run the 'Civil affairs in the occupied country – when we occupy them!' 'It is a much more amusing job than the one I went to in August & have just got out of. I have also just fired off my first address as Scientific Secretary to the Psycho Analysts so that I have been kept busy. I think it went down rather well – anyhow the place is improved beyond belief since we got rid of Glover & got Jones out of the Presidency into a sort of gilded shelf as "Past President".'

He was back at the King's Head when he wrote again to Vanessa on September 12, 1944:

> I have been down here for about 10 days & I go back to London on Thursday. You have never been here, so you would not appreciate all the changes but Karin came down here soon after the flying bombs started and has used the money we got out of the Army for damages while they occupied the house, for redecorating the whole place. The choice of colours was limited but out of the reds & blues & greens and yellows that they use for painting agricultural instruments, by mixing white with them she has been rather successful. Any how the whole place is very fresh & gay & looks in general rather like some foreign barge or fishing boat. The garden has gone completely wild with long grass & weeds growing everywhere & the trees which used to be clipped to form a thick hedge have shot up & separated into individuals. However all that can be put right as soon as we can get help with the gardening.
>
> The only thing that really matters is that one is not allowed to go out on the water. However I have a very comfortable lazy life. Karin has a patient staying in the house who is quite an amusing man & who, incidentally, can keep up our supplies of butter & eggs & so on owing to his connections with a London restaurant. She is giving him a rather intensive kind of treatment which takes 2 or 3 hours each day & I spend most of the day reading, or writing a sort of paper which is to be my first appearance as 'Scientific Secretary' of the Psycho Analytical Society or else walking about the fields & marshes. It almost seems as if the war was over here. We have lots of aeroplanes over us every now and then – I suppose on their way to Belgium or Germany – but if one does not go into a town one never sees a soldier which is a great relief. I shall be very glad to get out of khaki myself. . . .
>
> Love, Adrian.

The Council of the Society asked Adrian to recommend a painter for a portrait of Ernest Jones[82] now that he had retired from the presidency. 'Would Duncan do it?'

During Adrian's comings and goings he never ceased to write to me, except for brief meetings when we were both in London. In September, 1942, being pregnant, I had made that irresponsible and eventually disastrous decision to leave our ideal billet in Somerset and return to London.

Adrian and I occasionally met, sometimes in the flat or walking in Regent's Park. When he was in the mood he told me stories, sometimes about his family and their eccentricities, which he illustrated dramatically. There was one about his great-grandfather, James Pattle, who had died in India and been brought back to England in a barrel of spirits. During the voyage the spirits, or the corpse, expanded and when deposited in the hall, the barrel swelled, the lid burst off and James Pattle rose from the dead. This story has often been told but Adrian's version, as he rose, staring-eyed, white-faced, corpse-like, to his great height, must surely be the most authentic.

Once, when I asked him about analysis, he answered, 'You can't prove it by deduction.' My question was general, his reply specific. I asked what he meant, I don't remember what he said. My impression was of his caution, his implication that analysis was impossible to describe, or to be usefully discussed. (I even sensed that he had doubts about it as an effective treatment, specially for seriously ill patients, an impression confirmed when, in 1946, Dr Joan Malleson consulted him about me. He thought, she said, that I was not a suitable case for analysis. There he was wrong.)

I made him laugh, usually when I didn't mean to. For instance, I began solemnly to recite a poem by Marvell which seemed applicable to our situation.

Our love is of a birth as rare
As 'tis for object strange and high.

I got no further. He threw himself back in his chair, collapsing with laughter.

I discovered his love of music which Karin, because of her deafness, did not care for. My mother had given me records of Maggie Teyte singing French songs which I played over and over again. And there was a Strauss song, *Traum durch die Dämmerung*, sung by

[82] The painting is by Rodrigo Moynihan.

Elisabeth Schumann, which I connected with Adrian and his love of sailing. Whatever the actual words of the song it seemed to me to describe a boat on the water. The accompaniment is the water, the song the boat sailing on calm, gently rocking seas. Even then I couldn't be quiet but raised my head to speak till he hushed me. What he may have hoped for, always, was to get me to be quiet, receptive, briefly at peace.

For Adrian must, before long, have foreseen that I was heading for a major breakdown at some point in my increasingly disorganised life, which must have added to his responsibilities in the army, and his increasingly arduous work for the Society, worsened by Karin's prolonged bout of manic-depression. Nevertheless, he came to see me in the nursing home when our son, Robert, was born. And he visited me six months later at University College Hospital where I had undergone a radical operation. He came in surprisingly elated: 'I'm a great-uncle!' I couldn't understand his elation: 'You've got grandchildren?' 'Oh, yes,' he replied absently. Now I know the source of his pride and delight, his special feeling for Angelica, Duncan's daughter. When he left me he, characteristically, sought out my son Hamish who was in an amenity ward in the floor below, recovering from an appendix operation. He dimly remembers a tall man standing over him wearing an army mackintosh.

Adrian's war did come to an end – he had 'stuck it out' as he had doggedly determined to do. He was released in September, 1945. In October he and Karin moved to 1 Upper Harley Street where they lived for the rest of their lives.

18

DON'T TURN IT OFF, IT'S FASCINATING

The first time James and I saw Adrian in civilian clothes was in 1946 when he invited us to attend a meeting of the Union of Democratic Control in the Conway Hall, Red Lion Square. He had never lost touch with the UDC in spite of Karin's attempt to prize him out of it, as recorded in Virginia Woolf's diary. There were three other speakers on the platform, including Amabel Williams-Ellis. I have no memory of what was discussed except that they were considering the immediate post-war world and how democracy could be preserved.

Afterwards he drove us home, wearing his hat turned up in front like a sou'wester. We drove casually along Southampton Row and Woburn Place. James, equally casually, pointed out that we were on the wrong side of the road. 'There aren't many cars about at this time of night,' Adrian said, nonchalant as men who had begun driving before World War I tended to be.

Adrian and I met, formally, at one another's parties. And I went to tea with him and Karin. I made derisory remarks about my mother's hats. He turned on me: 'You're the last person to know!'

He continued to work till the last four months of his life, seeing patients attending meetings, editing the Journal, albeit with the help from Dr Willi Hoffer and Dr Clifford Scott, till, in September 1947, at his last recorded attendance, he resigned.

My cousin, Elizabeth Jane Howard, recalled a not very satisfactory experience when she encountered Adrian professionally:

> I went to see him only once, at his and his client's request. The client was a lover, and Stephen saw both me and his wife with whom I was great friends as Robert – the lover – was paranoid and extremely exhausting to be with and she was glad to share the load.

> Stephen practised on the top floor of a house in Regent's Park. He was, throughout the session, fairly hostile. I could see that he thought that Robert's neurosis sprang from his association with me. The session consisted of his asking me hostile questions which I remember answering as honestly as I could – at the same time feeling some dismay at his methods. It was my first encounter with a psychiatrist, and I remember thinking 'Gosh! I don't want to go in for any of this!' but Robert seemed to feel that Stephen helped him (although he did not persist with the treatment, so I suppose he cannot have been much helped). I compared notes with his wife afterwards – when she also had seen him, and her experience was much the same as mine. We formed the view that Stephen thought of us both (of women generally?) as a bit of a drawback.
>
> From subsequent experience of people in the profession I would say that either Stephen was not very good at it, or he found Robert a particularly devastating client. I remember him rather vaguely as being tall and handsome with some suspicion of vanity. But the feeling I had that he disliked me seems, in retrospect, distinctly unprofessional. He was not much of a sphinx so far as our meeting was concerned.

Gwenda David passed on a rather obscure account, told her by Karin, of a cruise he and she took towards the end of his life. His behaviour was so strange, and at times wild – he attempted to throw himself overboard – that the captain wanted them put ashore at Lisbon. But Karin vouched for his reasonable behaviour, assuring the captain that she would be responsible for him. The truth of this is confirmed by his daughter Ann: 'It was at the end,' she said, 'the very last resort.' She did not go further into this strange episode.

Dr Malcolm Pines, then aged eighteen, taking a medical degree in order to become a psychoanalyst, came to him for a training analysis. He remembers his gaunt figure, so often described, his bent shoulders, and his slow climb up to his consulting room on the top floor. He was obviously ill, but gave his illness no quarter. Whenever possible he chose to live in tall houses with tall windows – the King's Head was no exception. And, like most of his generation, he was impervious to cold. My only contact with him was through their dog and their maid Lottie. Supplies of horsemeat were hard to come by, but I found a shop where it could be bought, and delivered it down the area steps to Lottie's basement, which was well below street level, with small dark windows. I did not care for dogs; but thought this was a way to his heart. Above stairs, they probably never enquired where the precious meat came from.

In 1945 I had published my first novel, *When the Weather's Changing*, which I dedicated to him, and sent him a copy. After weeks passed without acknowledgement, I rang him up. 'What did you think of it?' With true Bloomsbury candour he replied, 'I don't think it quite comes off.' 'Oh, why not?' 'The characters are too much like bits of yourself.' This was the analyst speaking; and he was right.

I was passing the end of the lane that led to the back of the house where there were garages, and saw Adrian and Karin walking down arm in arm, his hat turned up in front as usual. For the first time I saw that he was an old man, or so it seemed then. They were an elderly couple, bound in easy familiarity by years of marriage.

On Good Friday, 1948, Karin asked me to see him; she was going out for a while. He was lying straight and unmoving under a white coverlet, expertly tucked in, his head propped up against pillows. The radio was on, where he couldn't reach it had he wanted to. Dismayed, I heard a religious service was being broadcast, part of the Christian liturgy for Good Friday, and I made to turn it off, supposing that he, like his famous atheist father, must find it tedious, if not offensive.

'No,' he said, 'don't turn it off. It's fascinating.'

So I sat by him holding his hand, while we went through the Seven Stations of the Cross, a lengthy proceeding. When it was over we stayed quiet and unmoving and peaceful. Then he said, as though faintly disturbed, 'The trouble is I see them crowding by the door, all my old friends.'

This is not to suggest that there was anything transcendental about either experience. His fascination with the service may have been professional, anthropological. As to his friends crowding by the door, had they not been in his mind always so that when Vanessa wrote of her intention to write about 'old Bloomsbury' he was able to reel off all the characters?

Adrian died on May 3, 1948, in his 65th year. Next day Karin wrote to Leonard Woolf:

> Adrian died last night in his sleep without suffering at all and not even knowing that it was the end. You know how I shall

> miss him but he had uraemia which is incurable and I am glad that he got away so easily. He was actually working though ill till the end of February.
>
> The funeral will be at Golders Green at 11-15 on Wednesday (no flowers). Don't feel you have to come but if you can and want to, do.

She wrote to him again on May 13, thanking him for writing about Adrian's death and trying to be at the funeral. She was 'missing him terribly' but was very glad to have work which 'helps me over'. After a long hold-up she was 'well away' with a book on Freud she was writing for the Hogarth Press, apologising for the delay and hoping that she would get on with it 'reasonably quickly'.

After Adrian's funeral Karin is reputed to have said cryptically to a friend: 'Even in this he has cheated me!'[83] Presumably she meant she would have liked to be the first to die. And to another: 'If only he had once told me he loved me!' But he did not love her. Nor, in the evidence of her letters to her mother, and from her behaviour, did she love him. But they respected one another, and worked closely together during the Society's Discussions; and with the years a deep affection grew up between them. He was at her side during her periods of depression; he never left her. And during his long, intermittent and final illness, she supported him.

She lived on for five years after his death, continued to work with patients and to see close friends, among them her ex-patient, Gwenda David, to whom she confided much of her disappointment and griefs.

Shortly after Adrian's death Karin and I met at Ann Synge's house in Paulton's Square. 'Now we can be friends,' she said in her straightforward way. I, bereft, guilty, confused, was nonplussed. But she took us on, introduced the family to the King's Head where we spent many holidays. Later, when I disparaged Karin, Janet, our daughter, remembered how much they liked her. At dinner, she entertained us with her wit and quick response, her literal interpretation of a chance remark. My reference to a 'hanging cupboard' took her into flights of macabre fantasy. James, who is terrified of mice, found one in his bed. It took Karin minutes to elicit the reason for his phobia: a middle-class Scottish boy, he had, it turned out, had field mice stuffed into his sporran by farmworkers during harvesting.

[83] Information from Dr Le Maré.

She liked to reminisce, and gave us a dramatic rendering of the Bryn Mawr rallying song, a loud, long, raucous cry augmented by a rhythmic tattoo on her throat. These stories were all about herself, but none the less good value. She described how, at a New Year's fancy-dress party, she had gone as Medusa with snakes in her hair, and reappeared on the first stroke of midnight wearing lilies, having been analysed. She took James sailing in their little open boat from Hamford Water to Harwich. Offshore it is very shallow, the wind blew up strongly and he shouted, 'We're grounding!' The sails were flapping wildly and she took no notice. She heard his third shout and raised the centre board, apologising: 'I'm sorry. I thought you said "drowning". *Grounding*, that's serious.'

When she cried, one evening, 'The Unconscious – don't touch the stuff! it's dynamite!' she was less than half-serious. She expressed the courage the early analysts had, exploring depths of the mind, their own and their patients', half-comprehending, aware of the damage that could be done, the pain that must inevitably be inflicted, the uncertain outcome.

With time, her depressions worsened, though we continued to visit the King's Head. Her manic flights were the more alarming; she crashed her Ford Anglia into a telegraph pole. And she made elaborate and costly plans to enlarge and renovate the King's Head, enlisting Mr Webb, the local builder, who, most likely, was wisely dilatory. She had been the innovator in her marriage, and it was possible to envisage how she carried Adrian along; also how his cautious restraint helped to keep her in check. But one scheme proved of extraordinary benefit to her family. I first heard of it as she came hurriedly round a corner with Mr Webb, carrying under her arm a bundle wrapped in straw. 'A mummified otter,' she explained. And went on to say that she and Mr Webb were going to renovate the cottages across the road. She had bought the land.

She and Mr Webb, between them, made a first-class job of the improvements; and the unoccupied cottages were taken as holiday homes at first, by Sir Basil Spence, the architect, Eduardo Paolozzi and John Hutton, who engraved a window in Coventry Cathedral – all with their families. The Hutton family lived there permanently.

Duncan Grant was Adrian's executor, and continued to administer the Stephen estate. In 1961 he 'allowed' Judith to occupy the King's Head – there seems to have been no formal agreement. This was the beginning of the Stephen–Synge–Henderson occupation. The family, children and grandchildren, returned to live in or holiday in the cottages, like the tide returning over the mud flats. Karin did not live to see the success of her venture. Beset with worsening depression, ill, bereft, she took her own life in December 1953.

On December 12, the analyst, Auguste Bonnard, wrote to Judith: 'I greatly admired both your parents for their courage, integrity and charm. When your father died I wrote to your mother saying what a noble person he had been. I had an especial occasion in mind when only he had the courage to speak out what was being held back in cowardly fashion by the rest. I can tell you that it made history in the Institute of Psychoanalysis for which I feel he was never sufficiently honoured.'

'Noble' is not a word he would have used about himself. Yet Karin used it in her diary when she was trying to define what perplexed her about his character. And Noel Olivier wrote of him as 'noble' in spite of her aversion for him.

In his obituary in the Society's Journal, Dr John Rickman came closest to defining Adrian's character: 'He was possessed of a kind of patient tolerance or acceptance of pain, and the work of living seemed to have set him free, more than most, to look with an open and unblinking stare on what was before him without being deflected by wish-fulfilment; he was supported by his genuine passion for the truth and by a certain satisfaction in debunking nonsense, dishonesty and pretentiousness.'

He will never be forgotten. Dr Malcolm Pines, who spotted a portrait of him by Duncan Grant in a gallery, combined with Pearl King to get the Council to buy the painting, which now hangs in the Council Room, a permanent reminder of this 'original, strange, spare and loveable man'.

Dr John Rickman's obituary in the *International Journal of Psychoanalysis* included the following tribute to Adrian Stephen:

> His contributions to psychoanalytic literature give little indication of his importance to the British Society. It was in conversation and in teaching he showed himself at his best, and next to that in the Council room. As he conceived it the British Society should be a free society of thinking people ... Without his persistence and characteristic fearlessness much less would have been accomplished in its reorganisation ... Uncomprimising as to the Truth, compassionate in personal relations, forgetful of self, his lonely path became a footway where others could the more easily tread.

APPENDIX I

ADRIAN STEPHEN AND THE CONTROVERSIAL DISCUSSIONS

After Hitler became German Chancellor in 1933 psychoanalysts in Berlin and Vienna began to leave, and in 1938, when Freud and his daughter Anna arrived to settle in London, they brought with them all those who were still at risk. These new arrivals brought with them ambivalence and downright hostility to Melanie Klein's theories, which were already opposed by some members of the British Society notably Edward Glover. He felt that she 'had gone too far' in her paper, 'The Psychogenesis of Manic-Depressive States' – she had dared to venture into the realm of the psychiatrist and to explore psychotic states and mechanisms in adults. Others, however, including John Rickman, Donald Winnicott and Ella Sharpe, read papers using the conceptual tools her paper had formulated.

Ernest Jones, who had been re-elected as President of the International Psychoanalytical Association, had become concerned about the divergences that were growing up between London and Vienna. Anna Freud pointed out that the acceptance of the Viennese analysts into the British Society meant that these differences had to be contained within the Society.

When Melanie Klein read her paper, 'Mourning and its Relation to Manic-Depressive States', the difficulties intensified. Her ideas began to be perceived by some as an alternative to the formulations of classic psychoanalysis, whereas she (Pearl King felt correctly) maintained that she was well grounded on Freud's contributions which she had extended and developed. Up to this point there had been widespread acceptance in the British Society of the view that Melanie Klein had made important and valuable contributions to child analysis which had extensive implications in the wider field of general theory and technique. This view was not shared by most of the Viennese psychoanalysts. The result was the consolidation of those supporting Melanie Klein who later became known as the 'Kleinian Group'. The uncommitted members of the British Society formed the 'Middle Group', to which Adrian and Karin Stephen eventually belonged.

Most analysts' concern was how they could contribute to dealing with panic and breakdown as a result of air-raids. Some members of the Society had grown angry over what they saw as the aloof and arrogant attitude of Ernest Jones and Edward Glover with regard to their relationship with other professional groups, specially the Tavistock Clinic with its eclectic approach to psychoanalysis. (The Clinic, established in 1920, was one of the first out-patient clinics in Great Britain to provide systematic major psychotherapy inspired by psychoanalytic theory for out-patients suffering from psychoneurosis and allied disorders and unable to afford professional fees (*Fifty Years of the Tavistock Clinic* by H. V. Dicks). Pearl King holds that there was fear of diluting the 'pure gold of psychoanalysis'! (Jones and Glover required a candidate for training to leave the Tavistock Clinic.)

Adrian Stephen deplored the lack of involvement of the Society's members in the war effort, whereas the Tavistock Clinic had been given the responsibility of organising Army psychiatry.

On the outbreak of war many analysts left London, though not Anna Freud, who organised a clinic for children disturbed by the London air-raids. But when some analysts, including Melanie Klein, returned in 1941, the discussions at the Society became increasingly acrimonious. Already in 1940, James Strachey, then editor of the *International Journal of Psychoanalysis*, wrote to Glover apropos the Training Committee meeting, which he could not attend as he was ill. 'If it comes to a show-down, I'm very strongly in favour of compromise at all costs. The trouble seems to be with extremism on both sides.' He wrote that Mrs Klein had made some highly important contributions to psychoanalysis but that it was absurd to make out they covered the whole subject and that their validity was 'axiomatic'. Equally it was ludicrous for Anna Freud to maintain that 'psychoanalysis is a game reserve' belonging to the Freud family and that Mrs Klein's theories were 'totally absurd'.

It became clear to Adrian, with his practical mind and lawyer's training, that the Scientific Discussions could not be usefully continued until the way the Society was run had been reorganised. Accordingly, after the Scientific Meeting in 1941, Adrian and Karin, with Barbara Low and Melitta Schmideberg, demanded that the Council call an Extraordinary Business Meeting to discuss the affairs of the Society. This meeting took place on February 25, 1942. The resolutions submitted for discussion concerned the discrepancy between Melanie Klein's approach to psychoanalysis and what was called 'Freudian psychoanalysis'. There was anxiety lest the appointment of officers, training analysts and the control of the Society should fall into the hands of one faction or the other.

Adrian's resolution was: 'That it is desirable that the rules of the Society be so altered that the continual re-election to office (other than the office of Honorary Treasurer) is rendered impossible.'

Adrian had long deplored the lack of democratic procedure. The controversies were discussed, month after month, at regular meetings. In spite of his involvements in the Army, Adrian only missed one. The stamina of the participants seems to have been inexhaustible but perhaps increasing bitterness reflected fatigue.

It was not until the Business Meeting held on June 26, 1944, after Edward Glover and Anna Freud had resigned office, that Adrian's original resolution, in a modified form, was proposed as a new Rule 6: 'No member who has served as President or Scientific Secretary for three years shall be elected to the same office until two further years have elapsed.'

This was passed without discussion. 'Complete victory,' Adrian told Vanessa. 'I have never fought a battle like that in my life before and I never dreamt it would be so successful.' It had all been 'great fun'. Adrian did not often express unqualified satisfaction over his own achievements!

The importance of the successful outcome of the Controversial Discussions is epitomised by Pearl King in her Conclusions in the massive record compiled by her and Riccardo Steiner (*The Freud-Klein Controversies 1941-45*). In his editorial comments Steiner said of Glover that, 'He of all the participants in the debate seemed to be out of touch with the historical reality and the institutional status of the British Psychoanalytical Society and of its future likely developments.' In her Conclusions, Pearl King wrote, 'When Glover, the Schmidebergs, Anna Freud and her Viennese colleagues withdrew from participation in the Second Series of Discussions of Scientific Differences, it was clear that "power" had passed to the pre-war members of the Society, augmented by the active participation of William Gillespie, John Bowlby, and Adrian Stephen, with Sylvia

Payne as Jones's deputy. (She became President following his retirement.)

'Compromise had been reached over training issues. From the point of view of Melanie Klein, this arrangement ensured that no other group in the Society would be able to interfere with her right to continue to make her own contributions to psychoanalysis.'

The compromise was the acceptance of three groups within the Society: Anna Freud, Melanie Klein and a middle group to which Adrian belonged. He favoured this compromise as did the Middle Group. He had played his part with his clear thinking, dedication and occasionally his happy use of simile, as the following examples disclose.

At the First Extraordinary Business Meeting, a resolution by Walter Schmideberg (about what is and what is not Freudian psychoanalysis) was not, in Adrian's view, relevant to the discussion. But Ernest Jones (in the chair) said it had to be discussed prior to any other discussion. Adrian riposted: 'Cannot agree to this. As well one could propose to discuss the distance of the earth from the sun.'

It was felt his own resolution on constitutional changes was not relevant to discussion on scientific matters. He replied: 'This, I think, is confusion of thought. The Society exists for scientific work . . . Improvements to the constitution are being brought forward in order to improve the conditions for scientific work . . . Alterations to the constitution therefore should be considered as being of scientific importance.'

Dr Glover, in a radio broadcast, had criticised the War Office Selections Boards in which Adrian was involved; and he amplified his disapproval in an interview in the popular magazine, *Cavalcade.* He had done this without consulting any other members and had given the impression he was expressing the Society's views. Some members felt what he had done was not illegitimate, and Adrian then made this point: 'Dr Glover may object to these tests, but he ought before he does find out what goes in these tests, whether they are not quite compatible with psychoanalysis. As far as I know they are in no way in conflict with psychoanalysis. . . . But the point is that Dr Glover does not know anything about it.'

APPENDIX II

CORRESPONDENCE BETWEEN ANN SYNGE AND LEONARD WOOLF

A. Synge to L.W.
June 3, 1964

Craigness,
Muchalls
Stonehaven
Kincardineshire

My dear Leonard,
I have just finished Vol. 3 of your autobiography. I have enjoyed it tremendously though I am not sure the method of digressions which you have used was a good one. But for me the fascination lies in seeing yet another aspect of all your semi-mythical people who surrounded us when we were young. Of course we saw you all in the streets and squares and even occasionally in houses but that wasn't how we knew you – I mean in the early 1920s – the real you and Virginia and Vanessa, Clive, Duncan, Roger and all of you were a compound of the gossip we picked up in the kitchen from such people as Daisy and her sisters, Lottie, Mrs Upp and so on. Of course they only referred to you as Mr W, Mrs B and so on and I can still remember how delighted I was when I first saw through this subterfuge. I said a compound and this material was compounded with talk from our own parents. Something seems to have gone wrong, there was always a touch of bitterness when mother spoke of the people you include in Bloomsbury and even father sometimes spoke in a tone which I took as a warning not to be deceived into thinking too highly of his family and their Bloomsbury

friends. I think Virginia was more or less excluded from the warning but why should I feel it? I also get the impression that there had been some sort of deliberate exclusion of our family from the magic circle and that they were trying to pretend to themselves that it was they who didn't want to be in it. Anyway, there you all were, larger than life, cracked up by the servants as 'great' men and women and played down by my parents as 'no more remarkable than anyone else for all they think so highly of themselves' and you were all a bit picturesque and awe-inspiring. I never asked any questions about why there should be this cold feeling. I don't think I really wanted to know the answer, it was bound to be a bit discreditable to someone. I know mother was a bit difficult but surely not so bad as all that in those days. Of course she was soured against art and literature by B.B. and Logan but she admired G. E. Moore as much as anyone and I have always thought psychology was much akin to literature so there was a possible bridge but it was never crossed. I'm not sure that I want to know the answer now but I thought you might be interested in the question and in how you all looked to us, aged about 6–8 I suppose. I say us but I'm not sure about Judith when I come to think about it, maybe I just mean me. It seems a waste, I was a quiet and affectionate child, a bit shy, but I would have been a good niece to you and Virginia if I had known you better & I felt rather short of relatives because, after the age of 5 or so I never really found the Stracheys congenial. It wasn't till much later that I got to know you for myself, much later from my point of view but only a little later from yours. You certainly have awakened a flood of reminiscence – what a mixed metaphor – but I thought you would like to know how much I enjoyed the book. I hope the next volume is well on the way but one day I suppose you will be dealing with people who are still alive and less interesting to me because not part of my childhood mythology.

I keep in mind that you lunch in London on a Tues. and have a mental note to get in touch with you if I should be in town on that day of the week but it is always another day – maybe one day it will be Tuesday, if so I'll let you know. Jane is much impressed by you but must feel as if you come out of the ark – she was saying the other day that of course

Maynard was getting pretty old by the time he wrote the General Theory & that accounted for some of its failings.

Yours, Ann.

L. Woolf to A. Synge
6 June 1964

My dear Ann,
It was very interesting to get your letter, which recalled many things to me almost forgotten. The trouble with Adrian (and later with Karin) was pretty complicated and dated from prehistoric childhood. Some of it is used in James in TO THE LIGHTHOUSE. 'Had there been an axe handy, a poker, or any weapon that would have gashed a hole in his father's breast and killed him, there and then, James would have seized it.' All Thoby's life and after his death his shadow lay over Adrian. Thoby was extraordinarily charming, physically, mentally, and in character. He was the sort of person whom everyone liked and many adored, and he was quite unspoilt by it. His father was one of his adorers; Adrian who was a rather peevish little boy annoyed his father. Adrian as a boy remained short, while Thoby and all other Stephens were magnificently tall. He became his mother's darling and outside the kind of inner circle of the three others. When he was about 14 or 15 he suddenly began to grow to his enormous height and I think this sapped his strength and energy. He came up to Cambridge towards the end of my time there; Thoby, who was immensely popular both in Trinity and Kings, had just gone down and the process of comparing the two which had done harm in their boyhood was repeated in Trinity.

When I came back from Ceylon, Thoby was dead and Adrian was living with Virginia in Fitzroy Square. Soon after she, he, I, Maynard, and Duncan set up a combined household in Brunswick Square. Adrian was extremely lethargic and critical. Unless pushed into it by Virginia or me, he rarely did anything but sit in a large armchair reading. He had a slight grudge against life, one felt, and he remained somewhat aloof and outside our circle which gradually developed into Bloomsbury. Then he fell in love with Noel and became still more passive, inert, depressed, and aloof when he was rejected by her. Then Karin fell in love with him and swept him into marriage. She was the exact opposite of him, full of energy, life, enthusiasm. She loved boisterous parties. She made up her mind that she would revolutionize him into the same kind of ebullient sociable person as herself. She could not of course succeed, and for a time she was, I think, pretty unhappy. The Bloomsbury mandarins, Vanessa, Virginia, Lytton, shook their heads over it, as you may imagine. They liked Karin, but in their habitual reserved way and with critical reservations. Adrian, as I have explained, had always been outside the inner circle and had resented it. Karin was not the kind of person to be able to bring him into it, and the war when they went off to live at Radlett (wasn't it?) increased the separation. After the war when we gradually all returned to Bloomsbury, they remained aloof and the situation which you saw as a child developed.

Virginia and I liked you and Judith very much and would have liked to see more of you. But you were extremely elusive. You would suddenly appear on our doorstep in Tavistock Square locked out from your own house and in need of food and shelter or Judith would come to lunch in Rodmell from a camp, but then you would disappear for months. But I must stop this. I hope I shall soon see you.

INDEX